SMART CITY—
BEING SMART

SMART CITY— BEING SMART

DR SONALI SARNOBAT

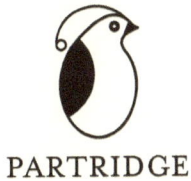

PARTRIDGE

To order additional copies of this book, contact
Partridge India
000 800 10062 62
orders.india@partridgepublishing.com

www.partridgepublishing.com/india

INDEX

SL NO	CONTENTS	PAGE NO

FOREWORD

BEING SMART

An artist by nature and a doctor by profession what am doing in this smart city issue?.

This was question asked by many. I always loved to explore and study different subjects. I was able to represent my city Belgavi in a seminar on SMART-CITY in Delhi, co-ordinated by Bhartiya streeshakti and National women commission. This fuelled my quest for more information and study on city planning as well smart development.

This book on smart city would be a simple guide to people who want to know what smart city is basically is! Smart city concept is actually being smart rather than building smart.

Kudos to the established government and Hon. Prime minister Modiji for this innovative effort. Hope people like this book. I would like to thank many who contributed in my effort to bring this book into reality.

May the smart city project be successful and we citizen get smarter!

Dr Sonali Sarnobat MD
+91-9632613269

1

SMART CITY OR A GLOBAL VILLAGE

It is necessary to understand that planning of cities is an ongoing process. Once a building or a bridge has been constructed and commissioned, the planners of those projects are deemed to have completed their work. However, the task of city planning never ends. Old buildings are demolished, new ones come up. New factories begin operations, new industries come into existence, some of them change, some go out of business. The number of people migrating to the cities may increase or decrease, traffic changes accordingly, business establishments undergo changes too. The quality and priority of services change, hence it becomes necessary to keep on improving administration and technology. The number of roads go up, they become broader; there are encroachments and they have to be removed. The number of schools, colleges, hospitals keeps rising; their requirements change. The administration has to keep a watchful eye on the entire city and its activities. Taxes have to be collected and taxation methods must be changed with the changing nature of transactions. Waste disposal has to be planned and its cost determined. New services have to be provided and old methods modernized. This necessitates assistance from various types of technical experts. After analyzing the available data, these experts assist the administration in formulating policies. Hence it is now recognized in most developed countries that planning of cities is an ongoing task.

Yet, we are stuck with the 20-year development plan mode. Our planning methods assume that there is no need for change in a city's plan for twenty years. That's the way we work. We think that the planners job is over once they have drawn up plans. However, this notion is erroneous and outdated. Planning is not a project but a process to be continually implemented in a city. We are also prey to the superstition that execution of a project according

1

to plan is everything. The Central Government has boldly taken up the "Smart City" project, however, underlying should not be the same half-baked ideology.

Cities change faster than the villages and hence the necessity to accommodate the change. Any shortcomings in the change need to be immediately addressed. There is a need to learn from the previous projects while planning the next ones. Earlier defects have to be avoided. New unplanned projects may need to be taken up at short notice. The economic as well as socio-cultural activities keep changing ceaselessly. New industries struggle to come up. People change too and strive for achievements. They try to adopt to the city and become 'smart'.

Imperialism which followed the industrial revolution ushered new technologies for comfort and spread throughout the world at an alarming pace. The nineteenth was a century of technological revolution. Cities like London and Manchester were living hell spawned by industrial revolution at the turn of that century. However, railway network assured food supply; trams, metros eased passenger traffic. Drinking water supply and underground drainage improved public health. The advent of city municipal bodies provided administration. Firefighters, Police and other law-enforcement agencies assured safety. The invention of electricity, gas and mineral oil fuels resulted in improvement in technology. Squalid localities were extinct. Cities shed their shabby appearance. Medicines were invented to combat Cholera, typhoid, Small pox. Anti-biotic were invented. The quality of civic life improved considerably due to the efforts of scientists and technologists. There was marked increase in life-expectancy. The new economy brought in new businesses, new skills, new industries. All this development had a favorable effect on the society and the economy. The ugly localities of London were transformed into a beautiful metropolis. With support from the King, Housman demolished the squalid districts of Paris and the splendid city came up. These city improvement techniques were followed around the world. Technical improvements, city planning methods and administration was undertaken in the cities in colonial nations too. Calcutta, Madras and Bombay were developed on similar lines by the British.

Machines, Technology and City Planning

A range of new generation of machines came up with new inventions. There was a steady growth of the use of machines and technology in the making of cities. City Planning and Development was combined in a holistic thought. Systematic thought was devoted to land, industry, civic localities and services and this led to rehabilitation of localities. The concept of beautiful garden cities became global and gave rise to planned improvement of cities. By the middle of twentieth century City Planning turned into an important sector of vocational education. In order to meet the demand of manpower necessary to provide holistic civic services, multidimensional vocational education became a part of curriculum in Universities. Cities became a field for research. This enabled cities in Europe to swiftly reconstruct after the destruction during the Second World War.

India attained independence in this era. This resulted in the severance of its connection to the administration, development and educational fields in Europe. As a result India was not introduced to the new developments in city planning methods. In 1960, the Government of Maharashtra enacted a law to determine the direction of City Planning. This resulted in increased involvement of the bureaucracy in City Planning, however ability and skills remained stagnated. The need for a large body of planners was not recognized. Not only was no research undertaken even systematic vocational education was not made available. Despite the stringent and complicated laws governing construction, the population in cities kept continually rising. This resulted in slums and quality of living in the cities suffered immensely.

Planning is a process, a skill just like cooking. If the management of a city is successful the city develops in a balanced way, if not, the development is off-balance.

At the turn of the twentieth century the issue of urbanization was seriously discussed in India. The subject had been researched, discussed, included in University syllabi and developed in Western countries immediately after the Second World War. However, India had remained incognizant of the worldwide research and the awareness of urban development issues. Research in hygiene, technology and architecture grew by leaps and bounds in India however, the study and education of city planning were ignored. The reason for this neglect was probably the general belief that India is a predominantly rural and agrarian country and will remain so in the near future. The need for economic planning had been acutely felt at that juncture but not for attention to the problems of urbanization. No one questioned the concept of a perpetual rural India. Even the need for study of urbanization and cities was not felt.

Resolve for Perpetual Development

The twenty first century brought with it new challenges of civic development on a global scale. It was realized that decline in ecology is a problem connected with urbanization. There is a general acknowledgement that unfettered consumption of natural resources have led to this predicament. The world became conscious of the necessity of sustainable urban growth. Efforts were made at the global level. The world ecological forum meet known as Rio de Janeiro Earth Summit in 1992 saw a resolve by the nations of the world for sustainable development. India was a party to this conference.

There was much talk about 'sustainable city' development in the first decade of the twenty first century. UN Habitat organization after studying the status and changes cities across the world developed an new method of study and planning of cities.

Awareness about the effect of development on air, water, land and people led to measures to address these issues. Older methods of city planning were discarded and efforts were made on a global scale to impart a new direction to development. Several countries like India from the third world were trying to emulate the western nations. They had no independent thinking and possessed neither the capacity not technology for research. However, they were also feeling the pressure for sustainable development.

Studies were conducted in several developed countries on sustainable city policies and many cities in small and large countries all over the world successfully implemented city planning policies. UN Habitat extended sizable financial and technical support for studying and developing ten cities in Maharashtra according to the newly developed methods. This planning method differed from the traditional planning method in its process of involving people from several strata. It involved explaining the process to the administrators and experts from various fields. However, in reality there was hardly any change in city planning and administration as far as perpetual city planning was concerned! Outdated policies based on old assumptions, erroneous planning schemes, faulty planning procedures and lapses in execution were carried over from the past.

Service, Management and JNURP*

The central government came up with the Jawaharlal Nehru Urban Rehabilitation Program in 2005. Seven years of execution of JNURP resulted in some progress in city planning process. From 2005 to 2012 the central government conducted this campaign to improve the basic infrastructure and their management. This involved four types of projects; two of these were meant for large cities and two projects were for small and medium cities. JNURP scheme, implemented in 65 large cities, aimed at improving basic civic services. Whereas BSUP (Basic Urban Services for Poor) aimed at providing basic amenities to slums.

The central government had chosen capitals of all states, cities above ten lakh population as well as religious and cities of tourist attraction. For all remaining small and medium cities UDSSIM (Urban Development and Services for Small & Medium Cities) was devised and for towns with minimum size and services INSUP was implemented. In all the central government was to extend twelve thousand crore for these schemes. The state government and local government bodies were also expected to invest in these projects in a certain proportion. The onus of suggesting projects helpful for city planning was on the local municipal bodies. Preference was to be given to projects for water supply, sewage and solid waste disposal. The centre was supposed to release funds only if the suggested projects were approved. For projects other than water supply and waste disposal, funds were to be released only if the state governments improved their administration. This campaign was of the 'stick and carrot' variety. Some states carried out necessary changes, whereas a progressive state like Maharashtra made a mere show of changes. Cities received the funds but very few projects were completed and even fewer were successful. The allotted funds in this scheme were not fully utilized as most municipal bodies lacked the capacity to manage the projects by appointing competent contractors, supervising the work and completing it within the timeframe.

The central government had promised financial aid on the condition that the state governments shall implement certain legal and administrative improvements. However, due to built in local and political limitations and indifference nothing much was achieved. No improvements came about in law, administration of planning. Some superficial changes were made. State governments and leaders in the cities did not attempt the necessary introspection. The "improvement project" opposite Thane railway station is probably a glaring example of this. This resulted in neither any improvement nor was the chaos around the station reduced. Sound pollution increased several times over instead of declining.

Smart City: Is it second part of JNURP?

The central government has announced the Smart City policy to tackle the old, suppurating problem of cities. The administrative process for this scheme is already afoot. The scheme to make a hundred Indian cities smart is being discussed all over the world. An important role has been assigned to the commissioners of civil service in large cities. In some cities attempts have been made to invite proposals from citizens. However, the response from people's representatives in the ruling parties is not very enthusiastic. It is difficult to judge how far they have understood the concept of 'smart'. The response from opposition ranges from blind opposition to 'let's see how it goes'. There seems to be no urgency and enthusiasm for study of the project. The JNURP had met with similar attitude. The centre comes up with schemes which the state governments and city administrations are supposed to execute. If a scheme is successful attempts are made to capitalize on it, if not the blame is transferred to the bureaucracy. This has been the general trend with all political parties. We will soon come to know what happens to the Smart City scheme.

BJP had included the Smart City plan in their 2014 election campaign. Most of their candidates had used it in their campaign without properly understanding the concept. While fulfilling its assurance the central government has assured financial aid to some cities from each important state. The first step of this scheme, namely selection of cities, was left to the state governments. Accordingly cities have been selected and applications from the cities have reached the centre. The central government has selected the first twenty cities in February 2016. Two cities from Maharashtra, Pune and Solapur have appeared in the list. Six cities from Karnataka also selected. Belagavi, My City is also selected which is indeed a proud moment. How this will affect the cities, whether it will have a bearing on politics, will there administration change for the better or worse or whether it will have no effect whatsoever is difficult to guess at this stage. All we know is the names of the twenty cities and the projected plans under the scheme. There's also news that political war is afoot in Pune on the Smart City project. However, information about the next stages of the scheme, timetable, names of companies to be given contracts, names of officers supervising the scheme and financial administration of the scheme is not yet available. Hence, it is difficult at the moment to make an assessment of the future of the scheme and its implications, though some companies (SPV) are formed.

What is certain is that Smart Cities have entered the imagination of citizens, and discussions in the mass-media. There is much curiosity among the public at large about the Smart City project. Hence it is necessary to respond to the interest generated among people.

The central government has included the condition of people's participation in the scheme and it still remains to educate and motivate people for participation. Some effort has been made with the available technology of smart phones and mass-media and objections have been raised against it too. The idea behind this book to educate people about the scheme to enable their informed participation. This response to the exigency of generating awareness is rather hurried. Later on there will be more time to review the process, take stock of things and discuss in detail. Let's now move to the main subject after this brief background discussion.

Knowing the Smart City

The broadcasting and communication media should play a major role to play in raising the level of consciousness of the general public. Unfortunately there is hardly ever a serious, informative discussion in our media. They lack maturity in terms of ideas, view points or analysis. It appears their main objective is to provide a platform for flippant political controversies. Hardly any space is devoted to issues of global consequence and various experiments. One gets the feeling that experts, scholars and researchers are invited for decorative purpose.

A book offers an opportunity to deal in some depth the concept of Smart as well as City and I hope readers will welcome it. The intention of this author is not to make hay while the Smart City sun is shining, but to provide more information and generate awareness among readers. It will be appropriate to begin with the basic concept of city for one may not be aware of the exact difference between a city and a village. It's an old belief that cities are not just bigger then villages in size but that they are smarter. Let's examine why this concept is correct.

Villages, Towns, Cities and Metropolis

City and citizens is a well-known pair of words, so is village and villager. People dwelling in the area which has the standard of a city are known as urban and those in villages as rural. However, city and village may be different they are not opposite meaning words. They are denoted by the words India and Bharat sometimes. Although there are contentious issues between rural and urban areas, their relation is inter-dependent. Neither can survive without the other. Citizens from both areas have an attraction to the other's environment. Villages supply vegetables, fruit, grains, water and several other commodities to cities. Whereas villages are dependent on cities for education, research, ideas, modern implements, machines, technology, knowledge, entertainment, market etc.

Villages are smaller areas living on natural resource-based occupations like agriculture, animal husbandry, fishing, mining. Whereas, cities are areas dependent on service and secondary occupations like trade, industry, transport, tourism, administrative and government offices, financial institutions etc. However, each country defines cities in its own way. In India, an area to be known as a city should have a minimum population of five thousand and population density of four hundred per square kilometer. Also the citizens must depend on non-agricultural occupations for their livelihood. There should exist an independent administrative body which provides civic amenities and collects taxes. In most of the developed nations towns with two thousand five hundred are considered as cities. In city an eighteen-year-old person is treated legally as an adult, but not in villages. Several towns with a large population are considered villages. Although towns with population in the range of thirty to seventy thousand have an urban look, Indians consider only cities like Mumbai, Pune, Nagpur, Delhi, Hyderabad as true cities. In reality and city or large locality is smarter than a village consisting of a couple of hundred houses. The reason is the variety found in those localities. A simple example is of a small locality which has no school since the number of children is not sufficient to start a school. The level of education is higher in a town than that of a village. Literacy is a mark of smartness among the modern societies. Cities which have a larger number of well trained, technically trained, skilled, highly educated, business people is considered smart. Since these localities have better trained and skilled personnel among their population, they can face and overcome challenges and calamities more efficiently. They can continue under duress for a long time too. This is seen in instances of natural disasters like earthquakes, storms, floods, famines; and they can quickly regain normalcy even in warlike situations or terrorist attacks.

However, this is not all that 'smart' involves. Persons who have many facets to their personality are recognized as smart as compared to others. Similarly cities have many characteristics. There is a wide range of variety of people, technical systems, societal systems, cultural diversity. This is why we can term cities smarter than villages. Similarly we can term metropolis as smarter than a smaller city.

Public Civil Space

I think 'for all' is the key word in the phrase 'Smart City for All'. In olden times cities always belonged to specific groups. The cities were organized accordingly. Common people lived in villages and seldom had contact with cities. Kings, nobles, generals, merchants inhabited cities. Places of worship belonging to various sects, temples, churches, mosques were located in cities. People belonging to these classes had the right to property. Cities would be protected by walls. Selected persons had access to cities. Travelers, strangers, soldiers, slaves or servants entered the cities. Women had no rights of any type. This arrangement has disappeared with the advent of democracy. Cities and urban populations have undergone sea-change during the last five hundred years.

Industrial revolution brought in its wake modern commercial and industrial cities. Democracy was born here. Paris and London are some examples. The populace at large gained democratic rights step by step due to the long drawn struggle by workers and women. Democracy as an ideal spread to the cities of Mumbai, Madras, Calcutta during the colonial rule and from there to the rest of the country. It was mainly the city dwellers who fought for the limited democratic rights to decide who should rule the land. Democratic institutions sprang up in cities during the colonial era. This is the greatest contribution by modern cities. Today every citizen enjoys the right to elect a representative. This is why we do not see monopoly of any particular class, religion, race or linguistic, cultural units in civic administration, and even if it arises at a specific juncture it does not last long.

It was in the modern cities that the thought of providing public civic service along with democratic rights. This led to the creation of network of basic technical services in each city. Basic civic services like water supply, sewage disposal and processing and solid waste management; fuel supply services like electricity, gas, petrol, diesel; communication network like postal, telephone and mobile services; civic food supply during periods of scarcity; primary education and health services; fire fighting services, police and security services; shops and markets; parks, gardens, playgrounds, theatres; zoos and museums; restaurants and hotels; affordable housing; hostels for students, women, disabled and the old came into existence in cities. These were public services and available to all. Everyone has free access to these institutions irrespective of caste, ethnicity, religion, gender. Some of these services are free whereas some are paid. It has been possible to provide electricity, gas, railway and bus transport on a large scale due to modern technology and management systems. Banks, lending institutions, financial institutions, satellites, institutes offering higher education, mass communication are considered public services. Not just the urban but rural population too has the right of access to these institutions. The spread of these services has turned into reality that these services should be available to everyone.

It is the existence of such public services and systems that has made the modern city very different from the cities of ancient times. Public utilities are still evolving around cities. Public welfare is considered as one of the most important function of the modern state. The entire society develops when the deprived sections are specially supported. It unifies the society. Conflicts, tensions, injustice, crime decline. The basic task of the municipality is to provide minimum public service to this end.

Unfortunately, at least in India, not much thought has been devoted to what constitutes "public". In an over-simplification, in the last few years public has been equated with government-owned services. For some time it was thought that such government-owned services should be available free of cost or at nominal cost to all. The railways are owned by the government, why pay fare? Water is available from nature free, why account for it? Why should citizens pay for water when it should be freely available to all? Some leaders of populist movements seem to be expressing such thoughts. That is why any increase in the rate of public services are deemed unfair and anti-people. Tax revisions, revisions of rates for services run by the government are thought to be a social injustice. Variegation in tax structures are thought of as social discrimination by some. At times people oppose modernization to improve service quality. The need for economy, financial management, accurate accounting is not understood. They find accounting and balance sheets meaningless. Economic illiteracy is to be blamed here. The ultimate losers are the poorest and deprived sections of the society.

From lack of financial literacy basic infrastructure services became a government monopoly in India, but little attention was paid to their economical management. Services begun in some cities could not be expanded as the maintenance, repairs took toll and capital could not be accumulated for starting new services. When crisis struck in 1990, it became essential to discipline on levels of government institutions. The process started at central government level. This was known as privatization, liberalization and globalization. The responsibility of some of the institutions from public sector was transferred to private sector. There was much opposition to the move without understanding the economic quandary the nation was in. Any participation by a non-governmental body was considered as privatization and opposed. The government services were considered sacrosanct and their losses were thought to be a saintly act. Privatization was equated with profit-mongering by propagandists.

In reality the move was aimed at freeing governmental services from the clutches of bureaucracy and politicians to improve their economy, management and efficiency. The policy meant involving non-governmental organizations in governmental work. The expected outcome was reducing the gap between public service institutions and the citizens and ensure co-ordination. It was aimed at making the municipalities more responsible. It was necessary to implement this change thoughtfully.

However, constructive and wide discussion became impossible due to fierce opposition. The bureaucracy and people's representatives turned privatization into opportunity for personal gain. The work was easily available to private firms who were willing to pay a bribe. The already corrupt municipal administrations became bribery ridden. An army of fake entrepreneurs, builders earning huge profits arose in every city municipal corporation. Reputed firms preferred to stay away from such contracts.

Privatization and liberalization was not an attempt meant to reduce the responsibility of the government but to render governmental service more effective. The central government planners and economists were aware that such an activity has to be handled with utmost care. Privatization has been attempted all over the world, in particular the formerly socialist block countries where the administration totally under control of the government collapsed suddenly, and is still being experimented with. Subsequently privatization was undertaken in a haphazard, hurried manner. Officials and people in power who were in a position to take disadvantage of the situation made full use of the opportunity to make money on the quiet. When privatization came to India the services offered under the central government improved markedly. Services in Passport, Income Tax, Customs became smoother, more efficient. The funds given by the central government was deposited straight into their bank accounts. The subsidies for ration, gas, education started being deposited into the bank accounts of the beneficiaries. The Adhaar card scheme was the mainstay for this service.

However, there has not been much improvement in the urban services. The people's representatives and bureaucracy in municipalities are averse to experts. They recklessly undertook privatization on their own which resulted in a distortion of the working of state and local governments. As a result several state level politicians gained from privatization. In every city a strong unholy alliance of private builders, contractors and local politicians came up. The politics of local lands gained key importance. Employment decreased and cities swelled in an unhealthy manner!

What is the main role of municipalities? Is it to create a monopoly of services or to administer effectively? It is important to discuss these issues at this juncture. Should municipalities create their own services or supervise the existing ones? How much should be the investment in services? How are the resources for this to be generated? What technologies should they employ?

How should the city be planned? How is it to be regulated? How should strict accounts be maintained? These are the questions each municipality have to face invariably.

My understanding of the Smart City Campaign is essentially making the public services of municipalities more effective and pro-people. If the citizens understand the importance of common interest their trust, participation and pressure on municipalities will increase. It is important that citizens not merely vote and demand their rights but also undertake responsibility. Only then can their conscious participation in keeping control over the administration, accounts and discipline be effective. Hence the necessity for each citizen to understand the concept of the Smart City.

A Smart World

One may recall that the idea of a global village was being widely discussed several years before the idea of Smart City was floated. The concept of a global village had the reference of information and speedy communication technology. In 2008 UNO declared that 40% of world's population lived in cities and the world was being urbanized rapidly in the twenty first century. It was after this in 2010 that the idea of Smart City came up.

Urbanization of the world will not mean an end of villages just as the agrarian revolution did not end animal husbandry or nomadic tribes, they continue to exist for thousand of years. Similarly villages and rural settlements will continue to exist even after wide-scale urbanization. May be their structure will not remain the same as it is today. In today's era of smart phones urbanization of families to some extent is already taking place in scattered small settlements and villages. Therefore the new era will not belong only to Smart Cities but to Smart Villages too. The social and economic gap will be considerably reduced between cities and villages. This picture is already visible in developed nations and might be seen in developing nations like India soon.

2

WHAT IS A SMART CITY?

I have arrived at the conclusion that 'Smart City' is an extraordinary concept to make the whole world a smart place. The advertisements in the media trying to explain the idea of smart city are emulating fantastical concepts of sci-fi stories. This is making the Smart City concept as daydreaming and impossible to achieve. Hence the requirement to explain the concept in a simple manner which the public at large can comprehend easily. In this attempt the information technology firms are in the lead. Let's consider some samples of their efforts.

This is the picture created by the IBM. No words are necessary to understand the three ideas in it depicted in blue and white symbols. The ideas can be presented in an equation:

$$\text{Smart World = Smart City + Smart Village =}$$
$$\text{Intelligent + Interconnected + Instrumental.}$$

Today there is a lot of talk of Smart City, but what we really need is a "Sustainable Smart City"!

Smart Cities

The advertisements generated by IBM and other companies are indeed attractive and easy to read and comprehend. They use common symbols and color pictures while presenting the idea in any language. They draw people's attention quickly and the necessary information and understanding flows to us. In these pictures the company has informed us of the important criteria essential for the creation of a smart world.

Let's examine the last component first, which is automation (machine intensive). We use numerous machines to reduce human labor and workload. The machine age has expanded considerably during the four hundred years since the industrial revolution. Agriculture, production and service sector related travel, commerce, goods transport and education, health - machines have gained importance in all sectors crucial for human survival. There is hardly any need to expand on this aspect.

The second component is that of the World, of linking the various cultures and machines to each other. The developing machine age connected the physical world through marine, land and air transport. Later telephone, and energy sources electricity and gas lines further connected people and lands. In today's smart world the satellites connecting through unseen waves are of key importance.

This communication system is the most important factor in a Smart City. A very ambitious project of collecting the information of every incidence, big or small, in the city and controlling the activities of the city through a control room is being run in some cities. The information technology company IBM has implemented a system in Rio de Janeiro using this concept. A conceptual picture is given below. This will help in understanding what can be achieved by a communications system.

Sensors of various types are installed at different points in the city. They are the eyes, ears and nose of the city. Information is relayed to the civic control room by these 'sense organs'. Cameras and sound detecting instruments continually monitor the city and are the artificial sense organs. Officers in the control room can view all the activities going on in the city. They immediately respond to any unusual occurrence, be it an accident, a traffic jam, crime in buildings, fights or sudden change in weather. The administration swings into action. Immediate, appropriate action is taken. Staff is alerted in the concerned area vide tv, mobile, radio or other suitable means. Concerned citizens are informed and alerted or put into action.

Various types of sensors are also implanted within each supply service too. Water and electricity pressure meters, instruments measuring the flow and gadgets fitted on underground water and drainage channels are interconnected. Instruments measuring difference in atmospheric pressure, wind, humidity, satellite pictures of clouds, rainfall, storms, geographical maps, details of buildings and traffic control signals continually feed important information to the control room. The information continually analyzed in the control room. Any significant changes, movements are scanned for probable activity and forecasts are made. The information is relayed to concerned systems, staff and citizens. Decisions are made quickly and action plans implemented.

On many occasions preventive actions can be taken well before the probable calamity strikes. For example, if the pressure in underground increases or water is blocked at some point the information arrives at the control point. Bursting of water pipes can be avoided. This reduces the chances of damage, resulting if avoiding inconvenience or accidents. Damage to man and material can be avoided. The sensors keeping a watch on the various activities and processes of the system are like the various instruments attached to a patient's body, continually monitoring movements and changes.

The instruments in this web keep the control room continually informed of each process and occurrence in the city. The city's services are controlled by analyzing the information received. Information technology companies are researching and developing such gadgets to manufacture and supply for use to city administrations.

Multinational corporations are on the lead in promoting the Smart City concept. Attractive advertisements, citations, incentives as well as propaganda, and pressure tactics are freely used by these companies to lure city administrations and political leaders. There is no doubt that the technologies have useful application. However, deciding on questions like whether a particular technology is useful to a particular city, is it truly necessary, what are the city's priorities, what and how much will the city gain from it, will the technology be too expensive, can the city afford it, what are the short- and long-term advantages and disadvantages, etc is of crucial importance and every city must search for its own answer. The task is not an easy given the highly competitive nature of today's world. It's like entering a luxurious hotel and deciding from the long menu what to order, how much to order, can one afford it, whether it is digestible, whether it is tasty etc. Sometimes cooking at home seems an easier option. Deciding on the Smart City technology is much more difficult for the welfare of a majority of the citizens is to be determined. It needs wisdom and foresight. Do our political leaders and city administrators have it in them? This is a valid question.

The success of the Smart City Project is dependent on the long- and short-term decision-making capacity of the city administration. The real problem is not of the Smart City Project but of the lack in discretion and vigilance of our administration! Cities are maintained well only if the municipal administration possesses wisdom. The administration which has the capacity for long-term planning is considered wise. When we come across well-maintained, smoothly running cities with beautiful environments one is pained at the thought of our own cities. Unless the civic services are managed well a city cannot become smart. Hence, effective city planning is the first step for a Smart City and here's where we are lacking. If we had any sense of planning our cities would not have been in such a bad shape. However, mere wisdom in planning is not sufficient. The administration needs to be wise too. We must ask what is intelligent administration. Creativity is very important in the age of information.

Will the world become smart if every city and village is made smart by use of modern technology? Necessary civic services will be available to all the people, but these services may not be all free. Space, time, proportion and affordability will determine the rates of usage of services. These might be termed 'variable rates'. Such a system is possible in the Smart Service age. The administrative apparatus will need to be perpetually wise and in dialogue. The idea is to create a network of geological services and invisible communication network for such smart places. Citizens are expected to receive effectively whatever service, instruments, knowledge and information they need, where they are.

This is a grand dream but it can come into existence. People are striving to this end all over the world. Attempts are being to involve the common man, to motivate him. Researchers in the field of information-computer-technology field think this achievable. Companies like IBM are on the forefront of this endeavor. RISCO, Siemens, Oracle and some other international companies are also leading in the field. But it is not just the giants who are active. Small and medium enterprises in many countries and imaginative individuals and also coming up with fresh concepts and contributing to the effort.

There is fierce competition to implement these ideas. Imaginative minds are colliding with each other, there is much interaction. Each concept is discussed threadbare, thrashed out. There is also co-operation along with competition. Not unlike the hybrids in living forms there are hybrids emerging in science, knowledge, technology sphere. An intellectual interaction process is unfolding. Machines and technologies are coming together, adopting to each other. New equipments with better applications are emerging. This is a natural, creative process of evolution and many times the silent evolution goes unnoticed.

The common man is attracted to the Smart technology, yet on the other hand there is doubt and worry. The reason being the dream of a smart world has not been accepted by all the people of the world. Some have refuted it, whereas some are worried about the competition and power of the multinationals. Some developed societies are ahead of the underdeveloped countries who have remained deprived from basic services or deprived classes in developing countries. Fear is also expressed that the Smart Cities will widen the gap between the haves and have-nots and between cities and villages. Whereas there is also the opinion that the cheaply available smart technology will narrow the gap. It is difficult to predict if there ever will be convergence in views, if at all.

The key concept in Smart City is of an all pervading, fast message system and linking everyone in the information net. Two decades ago the world had agreed on the concept of 'sustainable development'. Efforts were made to garner global support on this idea.

Sustainable and Smart Cities

Before proceeding with the concept of smart city in detail, it will be instructive to know about the efforts made by several cities around the world to implement the concept of sustainable cities. It was deemed necessary for every city administration to come up with targets and a timeline for each city depending on local environment, its economy, social structure and potential. In India a common administrative policy was evolved around 1960 as was the global trend then. Our efforts were in keeping with the prevalent concepts of city planning. It basically involved preparing maps of land use and regulation of the construction activity in the city by the municipality.

City planning has remained a mere technical formality. There is hardly any place for the city's geographical, economic, social, historical position and the specific needs of the people living there. On top of it, due to legal lapses, the municipalities are under no obligation to implement the planning. 'One size fits all' has been the rule and this has led to illegal, unchecked growth of cities which have now been authorized. To start with our laws governing city planning were utopian and impractical and led to disastrous consequences. Our cities are a victim of wrong prescription.

Much importance is laid on the necessity of full-fledged knowledge of local conditions, and full autonomy for planning and implementing schemes according to those conditions the local administration. The role of the municipality is of crucial importance. This necessitates a change in the administration. The municipal administration has to be ready and capable to make decisions independent of the state and national government. India has made changes to its constitution to this end.

It is very important that every city, its citizens, administration and people's representatives should be aware of which projects and what technology is needed by the city. Many a time inappropriate expensive gadgets are purchased in homes, offices and institutions and they remain unused. It is necessary to avoid such an error of judgment while planning for the smart city. The city administration also has to ascertain that it has the financial capacity to use the technology and keep it up to date. Trying to build the Smart City without proper financial resources can be an exercise in futility.

Smart Villages - Smart Cities

In the ensuing debate criticism has been leveled against Smart City that is a project merely to make selected cities smart. Questions are raised about the fate of other cities and mainly about villages. Is it not necessary to turn them smart too? These are valid questions. Here one needs to bear in mind that making certain cities smart does not necessarily mean depriving others from turning smart. Actually it is envisaged that when some cities turn smart other cities will follow suit. Villages are not to be totally ignored. Useful knowledge, technology and information is reaching villages through mobile phones, the internet, computers, cheap tablets and most importantly through the television. New, cheap and easy to use gadgets are making their way to the villages. Efforts are being made by governmental and non-governmental sectors to provide traffic, education, primary health services. India has been building a network of roads to transport products from cities to villages and vice versa. Urbanization has been influencing villages in various ways.

Therefore, there is no need to assume that villages will remain beyond or deprived of smart technology or gadgets. Many towns and villages will attempt to become smart whether it be with or without government aid. Actually, becoming smart with their own effort is the best and most effective way for any person or town. Self-motivated, self-disciplined villages and towns always succeed.

The lure of Smart City project is merely to motivate some cities. It is impossible to render such financial assistance to all cities and towns in India. Tonic given to some sick cities cannot become an ongoing measure. It is also wrong to assume that the sick, dying cities will be immediately rejuvenated. Efforts to that end are misleading. There could be several reasons why large cities with difficult problems have been chosen for the Smart City project. Just as rivers arise in hills and then flow to plains, newer ideas in human civilization arise in large cities and emulated elsewhere. This is the general rule of urban civilization. It is probably because citizens in larger cities are more open to experimentation. There is an urge to find solutions to old and new problems. These could be the probable reasons for choosing large cities for the Smart City experiment.

There is also an apprehension of losing something while gaining smartness. Older people and women are unable to appreciate the craze for smart phones, television and computers among the younger generation. In fact, they feel more importance is being given to machines than to humans.

There is also an consternation among certain social strata, local leaders and political parties in particular, of losing their rights. There is basis for their concern. The Smart City project envisaged participation of the administration and local populace, this is a probable cause for the discomfort among people's representatives.

It is a fact that the participation of local populace is restricted to voting in elections. People's representatives present civic issues according to their capacity, preference or will. Assurances are given to address them after election. It is possible to improve the political atmosphere and turning administration pro-people. Political leaders may be apprehensive of people discarding them. If a change occurs in today's narrow politics due to the Smart City project, it will be a welcome development. If they don't change they will be sidetracked. They are likely to be replaced with new, young, more democratic politicians. This may lead to political anarchy. Future is uncertain for sure.

Smart System - Smart Measurements

We attempted to understand the meaning and various aspects of the term smart. Today's technical-information-science age needs everything to be measured and calculated. Computerization has made it possible too. It is necessary to have some standards to measure smartness of cities and efforts are being made to this end. The discussion all over the world on Smart Cities has led to various definitions by people in an attempt to strictly measure and compare smartness.

It is possible to variously define wide concepts encompassing a range of interlinked elements. It is necessary to continue to discussion until consensus is reached. Various scholars are attempting to arrive at a meaning of Smart City concept within the premises of their chose field or city. Let us take a look at some of such definitions.

'When a city invests sizable human and social capital along with traditional and modern means of communication for its sustainable development and high quality of living standards; simultaneously prudently managing available natural resources; involves people in action programs, then it can be termed as smart.'

Two other scholars found eight facets of the Smart city common.

Smart administration, smart energy, smart buildings, smart transportation system, smart basic services, smart technology, smart health services and smart citizens are the eight important components of Smart Cities, say Frost and Khaliv (2014). This illuminates the eight facets of Smart City.

The 'National Institute of Urban Affairs' of Delhi has said in an article on Smart City that the 'machine to machine' principle should be used. This principle espouses decreased use of human interference in administration and making use of machines for administration instead. For example, the plans of a building should be submitted for approval to the municipal administration only through a computer. That the plan is in conformation of the norms laid down for the purpose should be verified by automated computers in various departments. The result should be reported by the computer system both to the applicant and the administrative officer. This will save time, reduce administrative interference and avoid corruption. Several such tasks can easily be performed by the modern computers and technology. There can be several examples of such machine to machine process.

3

SMART ADMINISTRATION

Various needs of each person, each family, each community and the widely spread industries-business organizations are dependent to a large extent on the public services provided by the city. In days of old tasks like preparing roads, digging wells, bringing water to the city through channels etc were undertaken by kings and lords. Rulers who provided these services were popular. These services were essential for transporting goods, trade and traffic. Octroi on merchandise was the chief source of income of the city administration. In addition, the main tasks of the city administration included taking care of external invasion, internal strife, crime control, social equilibrium and protecting life and property of citizens. This included construction of basic fortification.

Extension of modern civic services: During the last four or five centuries there has been a great increase in the number and types of services especially in cities and metropolitan areas. The most noticeable change has been in transportation field. Several options of conveyance have come up. Men and material is being transported by land, water and air routes. Roads have turned into conduits of several services. Drainage, sewage and water supply pipes run under, over or by the side of roads. Once electrical and telephone lines would run on pillars along the roads, now they are laid below the roads. Gas pipelines have recently joined them under the roads.

City Planning: Since the number of basic services has gone up, and since it is convenient to supply these from under the roads a great network of service channels has expanded beneath the roads. This enables activities on the land, in buildings to continue without interference by service network. Private or public institutions are involved in creating this service complex. Each service provider has a separate flow system, however, the responsibility to co-ordinate all services is with the city administration.

Roads in the city are owned and used publicly and the public utilities depend on their proper construction and maintenance. It will not be an exaggeration to state that the structures visible on the ground in cities is supported by the service network of water, telephone, electricity, currents running under the ground and the roads. Managing and maintaining the civic services has become an expensive and complicated affair. Considerable effort has to be invested in sorting out problems due to the expanding services of various types. The last couple of hundred years have seen a rise in capacity and technology to this end. Civic basic services has developed as a special commercial sector. The administration of every great city is dependent on the skills and technology of this sector. Separate departments have been founded in municipalities and corporations to handle this responsibility. Roads, water, sewage, traffic, buildings, finance departments are found in each municipality. Although these are organs of the same municipal body sometimes there is no co-ordination between them. It might be possible to form a department to co-ordinate central planning and action.

Administrative Structure: We are all too well aware of the shortcomings of our municipalities. They have various origins. They are like obstinate old maladies. Two of the defects I find very important. First is related to local politics and the second to financial indiscipline. Our representatives in the municipality do not appear to be capable, at least for the time being. Those who participate in local politics and get elected appear to be immature, semi-educated, and of feudal-rural mentality. They seem to have been elected by religious-caste-economic groupism. They do not think of the city's development owing to their immature politics and impractical political rivalry. They have little role in direct administration. The chief administrator or executive officer is not an employee of the municipality; they are servants of the state administration. Moreover, they are liable to transfer every three years. They do not necessarily bear a commitment to the city and the city's system.

This results in a tension between the municipal administration and publicly elected representative and the victims of this are the citizen. The role of citizens is limited to voting in elections and complaining about shortcomings in services. In short, the administrative system of our cities has become outdated and the challenge is to change it and make it modern.

To bring about such a change it is necessary to hand over all responsibility to the elected representatives. Just as a cabinet runs the state in independent cities the administration is run by elected representatives. This system exists in metropolitan cities like Delhi and Kolkata. However, our elected representatives have to bear no responsibility; they take credit for any good work done and blame the administration for any lapses. Due to this system the elected representatives do not take up any novel work nor do they allow the administrator to take it up. They want to exercise the right to financial management and decision-making but they do not contribute in any way to increase the revenue of the municipality.

Municipal administrators are usually very intelligent officers from the Indian Administrative Service. The Chief Officers of smaller cities are trained to handle administration. They are responsible officers and certainly possess financial wisdom. However, they do not have the freedom to take difficult decisions for the long-term welfare, financial development and sustainable development of the city. Since they do not have people's direct support they dare not take difficult decisions. On the other hand corporators with no financial training, wisdom or understanding take decision based on the criteria of political and personal gains which usually result end in damaging the city's interests. For example, the elected representatives never support the administration in reasonably revising the taxation rates to raise necessary funds. Administrators are rendered powerless against the elected representatives and succumb to their demands quietly. This renders the administration ineffective and loss to the city.

Information about the city: Information, sufficient and reliable about every aspect of the city, its citizens and departments is the basis of any small or large city administration. Information is essential for planning and implementing new schemes. Information is necessary for administrators to remain disciplined. Information is needed for efficient execution of any work in the city, for implementing and security measures. Information is needed for every kind of work. Some examples can make this point clear.

Even the demolition of an old, dilapidated, dangerous, two-storeyed structure needs a lot of information, even if the building is unoccupied. Information is needed as to whether the structure is wooden or brick, what is the roof made of, the number of doors and windows and the material they are made of, how are glass structures to be removed, where are they to be stored, what is the number of wires, pipes, tiles and how can they be reused is to be assessed. After all the information is collated, what material of the salvage can be resold, how much will it fetch, how will it be extracted, how many labourers will be necessary, where should the discarded material like stones, bricks, soil be stored, how are they to be transported, what security measures need to be taken is to be planned. If the demolition is on private land care needs to be taken that public services are not disturbed and permission needs to be obtained from the municipal authorities. Such a permission can only be granted on the basis of information. Much more information is required for construction of new buildings and demolition of old structures if they are public places.

A large amount of information is needed for security and safety measures to be incorporated in the city. In case of floods, where and what quantity of water will flow has to be assessed and provision is to be made for speedy drain of accumulated water. Lapse on this count can disrupt several other services like electricity, traffic etc. The number of accidents can go up at such times. Vehicles and hospitals have to be in a state of readiness to handle such situations. Fire-fighting service, ambulances should be all set. Various types of natural calamities can strike. Landslides can occur. We have witnessed the extreme hardship the citizens of Chennai had to face in the recent floods in that city.

There was a deluge on 26th July 2005 in Mumbai and the haunting memories of the calamity are still fresh. Meteorology department of the government plays a vary important role in such situations. Although innumerable efforts have been made to predict floods and quakes, famines and droughts and there have been advances made the uncertainty in their occurrence still looms large. The dangers will be multiplied many times over in the scenario of changing climate. The task remains two-fold safeguard cities on one hand and alerting the citizens on the other.

The Japanese are exemplary regarding information about earthquakes, construction techniques and citizen alertness. Such system is hard to find in any other country in the world. Luckily, such information can be available to everyone in the world today. Technology has been developed, and is being developed to meet these needs. Every city can contribute to this end. A gigantic store of information can be available to all cities in the world. This shall be a treasure for generations to come. Collating such information, comfortable exchange of information with others and quickly relaying necessary information to those who need it are aspects of Smart City and they will continue to grow. It is not for nothing that the present age is known as the age of information. Making the benefits of this age of information to all citizens is becoming a city with smart information. People in our country have recently gained the right to information. Today this information can be accessed with some effort by applying to the government. However, the object of the Smart City is to make whatever information one needs without asking for it in an easy and transparent way. The foundation stone for the right to information of the Smart City has been laid down today, constructing a multi-storied structure on this foundation is a continuous process.

Civic Law, Rules and Implementation

It is necessary that citizens understand the laws in a simple, easy manner. These laws should enumerate the responsibilities of the municipality, the duties of the citizens, rules governing development and construction of buildings as well as laws governing taxes and service charges. Based on these laws each municipality can formulate rules and make amendments.

Our administrative structure visualizes autonomous municipal bodies, however, there is much confusion in this regard in reality.

The issues faced by small and large cities in this connection are quite different. For example, smaller towns have limited sources of income. Land and land revenue is considered the main source of income for the municipality, but the tax on non-agricultural urban land is collected by the state government and the property tax on buildings goes to the municipality. These are to be assessed every three years by law and used to be assessed as such during the British era. However, most of the municipalities have not done so during the last thirty or forty years.

If there is no coordination between the state government and the municipalities regarding the laws and their implementation, if not only affects the city but the citizens too.

Laws governing construction of buildings are so complicated that it is difficult even to decipher these which results in misuse by some elements. Several organizations are involved in governing one aspect and there is no coordination among them. When flyovers are constructed disputes arise as to whom the underlying space belongs to. So many organizations are digging roads in the city that even the municipality is unaware of the activity. Some footpaths are in the jurisdiction of one organization while some are with some other organization. For example if the corporation constructs roads in an industrial area there is dispute with the municipality as to who has to carry out maintenance on these roads. If a government body undertakes a housing project, the municipality does not provide water connection for there is no coordination. Several times developers get private roads constructed at government expense due to these gaps.

The spheres of responsibility of the railways, municipalities and other government bodies are not clearly demarcated. This results in disruption in the city and citizens suffer.

Several times it has been seen that officially sanctioned buildings have difficulty in securing a water connection whereas unauthorized structures get connections.

The central government provide funds for the Smart City project but unless there is an effective mechanism to sort out numerous difficulties regarding laws and rules, take firm decisions and controlling the bureaucrats and people with influence, it will be impossible to turn cities smart. If people and their organizations approach courts all efforts will be in vain. The legal difficulties remain to be addressed as of today.

The biggest hurdle in improving cities is that of the government mechanism. Provision has been made of creating a 'special purpose vehicle' or SPV organization to surmount this difficulty. At present such organizations have been operating on state level. The step is new in municipal sphere. However, there are some doubts about this as yet. It is not a fool-proof solution but a practical measure. How far it will succeed is difficult to gauge at present.

If political forces, parties and leaders approach courts against SPVs all work will come to a standstill. We are yet to know what solutions have been found to counter such legal difficulties. It will certainly be a smart step to anticipate the probable difficulties and find solutions for them.

Smart Energy

The most important topics in connection with the discussion on Smart City in developed countries is around non-conventional energy the adverse effect on the environment due to conventional energy sources. Electricity consumption has multiplied several times over in the last few decades. Special efforts are afoot to save electricity and employ smart technology to bring precision in electrical consumption. A time-bound program has been chalked out by most countries and cities to save electricity. For example, an organization in Italy aims to save 40% electricity by making streetlights available where necessary on the roads at night and at specific locations only.

Several measures are being employed in Europe and United States to save energy in transport. Roads are being recreated with special place for pedestrians and cyclists. In Berlin and Copenhagen cities several hundred kilo meters of cycling tracks have been created as incentive for people to use them. Policies covering energy use and pollution have led to restrictions on private vehicles. In some cities the plan envisages use of only electrical operated vehicles instead of the ones running on petrol and diesel. Several restrictions are being imposed on private vehicles. Such efforts for smart energy will prove very useful for all the cities world over. This is expected to bring about a revolution in the public services. In some cities in India, measures have been taken to save electricity. The streetlights come up automatically when there is no sunlight and shut down when there is sunlight. Streetlights can no more been seen in Thane now during the day. Incentives are being provide to use solar power and use of LED bulbs to reduce electrical consumption. If municipalities apply their minds to the smart technology of generating methane gas from biological waste they can tackle all three issues of waste disposal, environment damage and energy consumption.

Building and Construction

Smart construction includes houses, factories and all sorts of large or small, private or governmental building and construction of basic infrastructure. Smart construction includes design, planning, drawing, construction and maintenance of buildings. Choice of building material is also included in it and also methods of saving on space, energy, water, cement-steel, metals and time. In addition it encompasses safety of workers and prevention of nuisance regarding dust, sound, transportation etc during construction. This special field of eco-friendly construction is a recent development. Importance is given to recycling of water and automated control of non-conventional and conventional energy. Sunlight, temperature of exterior weather, wind are noted and the interior of the buildings is maintained automatically with the use of computers. Specific parameters have been evolved for such smart buildings. Older structures in the city can also be rendered smart using technology. City administrations are issuing certificates for smart construction.

Smart construction methods being generally employed in developed countries, have not evolved in a year or so. Everyone from the top executive to the lowest level worker everyone has to be trained in the use of this technology. Mechanisms are developed so that no one far or near the construction site suffers from dust or noise pollution and accidents. Workers are not only insured, but severe and immediate punishments are administered to those responsible for accidents. Reasons for accidents are searched and workers are trained to avoid repetition of the underlying factors.

The essence of smart construction lies not just in erection of buildings, roads, bridges and all sorts of grand and complicated structures but also in systematic, safe and quick demolition of old buildings and bridges and in maintenance and repairs. Readers will realize the extent of progress we have yet to make in the construction sector. We can successfully employ Smart City project only if we start training workers in construction industry and provide for safety measures. It is necessary to smartly construct in a timely fashion and not enough to merely build smart looking structures If these objectives are not incorporated, cities can not be said to be smart. Turning wide-spread sprawling slums into neat, sanitary living areas and providing the poorest of the poor with shelters consisting of minimum facilities is what Smart Cities are about. Special construction technology will have to be developed to this end. City space and time will have to be planned in minute detail. The most important aspect of smart construction is planning the city smartly with transparency and involvement of citizens.

Transport System

Transport system in cities, in particular the metropolises, has turned out to be a vast and complicated subject. The problem is of urban environment further complicated by political ignorance and financial and administrative confusion. We have arrived at this difficult situation not only because of increase vehicular or human population, but because of a total lack of urban traffic policy.

When there were no private motor vehicles in 19ᵗʰ century London, chaotic traffic had turned into a public health hazard. Then arrived vehicles running on rails. Over a period of time metro rails were laid under the ground and traffic on a large scale began underground in a systematic way. The roads became unclogged and people breathed a sigh of relief. A state of discipline was established and chaos on the roads was reduced. Technology assured large scale and fast traffic system and several traffic-related problems were handled in next 50-75 years. However, the number of private motor vehicles grew considerably after 1960 in all developed nations. Motor vehicles took centre stage in the traffic policy. The steep rise in pricing by oil producing countries in 1970s was a big jolt. Curbs were imposed on privately owned motor vehicles in Europe to restrict their numbers. Singapore adopted these measures and made its public transport system very effective by curbing private motor vehicles by imposing financial restrictions. In the United States, however, public transport and bicycle use is encouraged and alarm raised by futuristic experts is being ignored.

Heavy fines, expensive parking and strict punishment to traffic offenders are effective measures to control private vehicles. They are the best measures to make traffic smart. Their success and usefulness has been proved in most cities. In the recent odd-even number vehicle rule the indisciplined vehicle owner had to pay a fine of two thousand rupees. This sorted out even the arrogant, rich, careless of drivers. Public instruction, advertisement and use of various communication media are effective ways of making traffic smart.

It is also necessary to encourage pedestrians and cyclists in smart traffic system. A major problem in India is the fast motor bikes being used by young people. They treat all traffic rules as obstacles. One can witness gangs of three or four youngsters driving recklessly and blowing horns at any time of day or night. They drive on footpaths endangering the lives of many.

Basic Services: Water, Sewage, Drainage processing, Recycling and Solid Waste Management

It is impossible to review all these systems in detail here. Water supply, sewage and solid waste management are very important service for every citizen. The difficulty is that it is not possible to measure the smartness of each of these services in numbers and figures. For example, to understand whether a city is smart in water supply it may be possible to measure how many liters of water is supplied on an average per person, per day, per month and per year, but it is also necessary to know if everyone receives it in equal proportion or what is the extent of leakage, or whether it is pure and potable, whether it contains minerals, is it affordable and whether citizens pay for it on time etc. It remains to be seen whether criteria for all these parameters can be fixed in a scientific manner using smart technical systems. As of now it has not been possible to measure everything in terms of figures, one hopes it can happen in future.

Most cities in developed countries are already smart in respect of water supply. The instruments may not be using the latest technology always, yet one can say that the water supply system there is very efficient, which means all the people in cities receive a calculated supply of sufficient, reliable and clean water and charges are collected from citizens for use. Leakage and theft is very low, say 4 to 10% only. In our cities this percentage is anywhere from 30 to 50%. In developed countries the recovery for water charges is between 90 to 95%, whereas in our cities this percentage is between 50 to 75%. Our water management suffers from a three-fold problem - low rates, pilferage and insufficient payment of bills. All this is true, yet this is not the only problem. In cities in desert lands like Dubai and Tel Aviv although there does not exist a source of sufficient natural potable water it is supplied to citizens using technology. Hence, the real problem in India is of technical and administrative backwardness. Citizens may be victims of mismanagement, but they are also contributing to the financial sins. We are ignorant and cunning. Water in cities is available to the rich at low and to the poor at high rate. We cannot deny this reality. Leaders and movements claiming to champion the interests of the poor have also been found opposing any improvement in water management. All sorts of movements in cities, genuine or otherwise, follow them and oppose improvement in the system. Owing to such indisciplined and irresponsible attitude almost all cities in India are in a grave crisis in water supply and sewage. The situation is complicated by our social makeup, politics, extreme disparity and traditional discrimination. In fact there is no need to discriminate between urban and rural water supply. Similarly, the competition between demand for water for agricultural use, industrial use, commercial use and domestic use is also detrimental to water management. We cannot truly afford to remain so backward in this era of Smart Cities in the twentieth century.

It can be proved with the help of statistics that water is available in sufficient quantity for the future too. However, we do not have statistics readily available about how each social group uses water, how many people use water for washing vehicles, how many people in poor localities have to travel what distance to fetch water, how many receive water by tap, what is the attitude in using water, how many pay the administration regularly. Although some statistics may available about water usage in cities, it does not reflect the extreme social disparity in averaged figures. The only figures available from the municipality are about domestic and commercial use of water, that too because the rates charged are four to five times higher for commercial use than those for domestic use. If we want to make the city smart all factors large and small should be measurable accurately at low cost. They should be accounted and balance sheet drawn. Leakage, pilferage, corruption, negligence should be located and its quantum ascertained. Also must be ascertained whether citizens using the water are paying for it properly in time. Unless timely maintenance of the water system and other managerial aspects can be checked minutely, water supply will not become smart, and it is most important that it be smart is a pre-condition. Moreover, when it is seen that all citizens are receiving this information, understanding its importance and their water consumption is responsible only then can we say that water supply is smart. If this happens we can say we are a step forward towards Smart City. Two-panged plunder by private and government bodies of valuable and scarce water undermines sustainable development.

Citizens and administrations in metropolises in developed countries are seen to be water-literate. If we compare our water supply with theirs, every city can measure how smart is its water supply system. This will enable to take action based on which aspects need to be improved. We must understand that smart water is a necessary process for each locality to become smart. This is known as 'bench-marking'. Which, in other terms, is deciding on the minimum requirements and comparing the actual water system in each city with it.

The water supply system in Singapore is very effective, efficient and co-ordinate in most aspects mentioned above. It is truly smart. Like electrical use the extent of water use determines more or less smartness, this is treated as just there. A mere 4-5 decades ago this little country was dependent on Malaysia for its water requirement. By strict planning and inventing several ways to reuse water it has now become self-sufficient. That low and equal rates are unjust is a principle accepted there long ago. 40 liters of water is given free to every person and for use above that water has to be bought at an increasing rate. The attitude to co-operate with the government has been inculcated among citizens there. All this has happened much before the talk of Smart City came into vogue. Since the foundation has already been laid, it will be easy to acquire further technology for smart water management. For example, a technique to collect information and a mechanism to instantly transfer it to computers is easy to implement there. It will be easy to accurately calculate and analyze data being continually received. This information can be utilized for more efficient water supply. Space satellites, computers and mobile phone technology can be easily used to make the system smarter. It is also possible by smart technology to receive payment from the client's credit card. However, smart water will be a challenge in small and large of our cities where the municipality is supplying water but there are not meters to measure outflow, pilferage and leakage are rampant, waterlines are old and repairs and maintenance insufficient and administrative corruption and petty politics hold sway. It might be easy to provide smart water in cities where there is no water supply or where new water supply system is being created.

Smart water supply is an important feature of a Smart City, however, this requires great political and administrative will to implement. One encouraging feature is that the financial investment or burden is not very heavy. The difficult part is civic and social education. Even more difficult are the issues connected with environment and natural water sources. To further complicate the task are problems regarding estimates of available natural water, technical planning capacity and administrative implementation. The biggest challenge is the need of various geological and administrative departments working together and co-operating whole heartedly. Smart water is closely linked to financial policy regarding water. A misconception has taken root during the last sixty years or so, namely, that providing water at a flat rate to all is in keeping with social justice. Various social groups have popularized it through agitations. Many municipalities are financially burdened with this so-called economic equality.

Financially strengthening the public water system is a need of all habitations. A completely new, improved system of just distribution of water needs to be brought in. The object of smart water distribution is to fix a meter on each connection and supply water by telescopic method in a transparent way. However, the complicated water-maths needs to be explained to each individual and each social group. Agitators have been opposing change out of fear that privatization will make water costlier. There is an underlying financial and water illiteracy to the traditional, socialist opposition. There is no doubt about their concern for the poor, but most political parties today have taken up the points from their campaigns and are misusing them to protect self-interest by creating a specter of price-rise. Social damage is the result when, genuine and sham, both types of leaders take up the same path. When collective power is misused in this manner, it is the public services which suffer. Whether it is the public water for distribution in cities or for from dams and canals supplied to agriculture when mobbism is resorted to by selfish mentality it takes a toll on public interest.

Today even the poorest of poor families owns a mobile phone. If all consumers can receive details of their water consumption and charges through mobile message, they can check it themselves. They can complain about if there is any discrepancy. We get details of bills for various services on the mobile - electricity bill, phone and mobile bills. We get bills of water or other civic services and taxes on mobile. But we have remained backward regarding local or essential services. We must aim to spread smart city technology to every city, town and village level. People need to be educated and convinced against the resistance to smart services.

There are various groups opposing smart water schemes. One is of people's representatives, another is the tanker lobby. A third one is of mediators who provided unauthorized connections to the poor in slums. However, it is not that these problems exist in cities which have enough water supply. There are several districts, talukas and towns which are suffering from lack of water due to insufficient water, low and unreliable rainfall, and lack of investment in water projects. It is sad that there are strifes and politics surrounding water. This leads to the extreme thought that the water management system should be freed from the hold of political and social movements and handed over to technicians, scientists and financial and administrative experts.

We need to understand that our social and cultural burden is breaking the back of basic service like water supply.

Decisions about basic services in many cities have been taken based on political, social and cultural grounds rather than on sound and objective technical and financial criteria. This has led to discrimination between various social groups. Strife and clash of interests arises between social groups, the minority, poor and Dalit localities are affected in particular. They remain neglected. It is possible to study this socio-cultural reality and provide the benefit of basic services to everyone. Appropriate technology and management systems can be adapted if one has a vision of social justice. It is very important and easily possible by involving people, gaining their trust and by using smart technology. However, political hindrances will have to be removed while implementing smart technology and with transparent, inclusive policy. This involves educating the political leadership which in turn depends on an educated public. It is also true that if the leaders really desire to good to the people they can educate them. Creating smart citizens and smart leadership can not be done by technology but by smart education. This will involve an improvement in the educational field. This is no easy task. In our vast, diverse land divided by inequality it is a hundred times more difficult than any other country.

At this point, we can not go deeper into the subject of water-related other services like drainage and sewage. However, what one can definitely say is that the service charges for this basic service are extremely low.

As far as solid waste management is concerned Indians do not pay any charges to any municipality for this service. We ignore the rules and do not bifurcate the solid waste. Most citizens do not think it is their responsibility. When even the highly educated and rich citizens in our cities are not as concerned about their responsibilities as they are of their rights and privileges, what can one say of the rural, illiterate and poor citizens. In reality, it is a universal observation that the richer strata of the population which generates the most solid waste.

Democracy has filtered only to the level of elections in India. If we want it to percolate further down and strengthen it for development, 'smart and sustainable water' will be the most important policy. Hence, people in all cities should support this policy knowingly and with proper understanding.

Dialogue and Information Technology

We have become accustomed to all sorts of machines and electrical gadgets. Mixers, fans, fridges, tvs, and motorbikes have pervaded every home in cities. Mobiles and smart phones are latest examples. We have been using various gadgets for decades now.

Newer, cheap, attractive, smart, easy to uses gadgets are entering the marketplace to help us overcome our laziness and make our work easy and fast. Intelligent people assess needs and human nature and invent them. Then they are marketed by use of attractive advertisement campaigns. From electronic watches to computers, simple phone to complicated gadgets like tablets are being made available to public. The Smart City thought can be spread wide when citizens possess such smart technology.

Smart gadgets can help in avoiding wastage or minimize the use of costly resources. For example, holding the hand under the tap starts the water flow and removing the hand stops it. Electricity is saved when locking the front door of the home or office automatically results in switching off the lights and fans etc in the building. This field is ever developing. The Smart City policy will entail averting crime or accidents.

Lamps on our streets continue to be lighted even after sunrise. When we forget to switch off the pump supplying water to the water tank on the terrace, we waste both electricity and water. Taps in the toilets in government buildings are found to be leaky many a times. We see such irresponsible public behavior in our governmental and institutional sphere. The reason is, of course, most of our population has irresponsible attitude and behavior. Such behavior results in waste of public fund and resources. The gadgets and controlling systems used to regulate such behavior have technologically developed to a great extent in the past hundred odd years. Saving money is an important aspect of commercial setup. Commercial establishments employ money-saving devices continually. When the occupier of a hotel room lifts the key from its socket while leaving the lights, fans, tv, geyser and air-conditioner etc are switched off automatically. This saves electricity irrespective of whether the client is careless or not. However, governmental organizations are always lacking in taking up such measures. Municipalities do not appear conscious about using the several smart techniques now available to save power in street lighting. We often hear complaints about lack of funds but there is no effort to account for wastage of resources. Smart technology is now available to save money, water, electricity, labor and time. Such smart, quick and automatically accounting of resources should be employed in administrations in a major way. This can be achieved through constantly updating programs.

Health Services

Public health services have expanded considerably in modern times. It is considered as one of the important tasks of a government. These include primary health services to citizen and disease prevention. Communicable diseases are kept under check in a major manner by such government services. Prevention of infant mortality and taking care of women's health are two major responsibilities of the local administration in our poor and half-literate society. However, our municipalities are not very efficient in providing these services. Houses, water and sewage systems are not available in adequate numbers for the migrating population in our metropolises. Such a population is not very health-conscious for they are not educated enough. Public health service can be rendered smart with the help of other services and governmental health organizations. There is a dearth of public toilets, washrooms, primary health centers and trained staff to man these. Although plague and smallpox has been curbed to a large extent, T.B., cholera, typhoid and malaria have not come under total control since the sewage, solid waste management and public toilet systems are lagging.

There is a lot of discussion at global level about smart health services. However, the requirements of various social groups are different from the problems in our cities and there is not much discussion about these in our deliberations.

Educated public opinion is an important aspect under Smart City and it is related to smart citizenship. This aspect has been discussed below. Smart health services are for public health and public health is not possible without smart citizenship. Civic administration will have to take these factors into consideration while planning smart health policies.

4

CITIZENS

The qualifications for smart citizenship is literacy and minimum school-level education. In developed countries all the citizens are literate. In our country, education level is higher in urban areas but lower in the rural areas. Moreover, the quality of education is a major problem. Hence, although it may not be necessary in developed in other countries, in our country smart education is a necessary aspect of creating smart citizens.

For cities to be smart all their citizens need to be sensible. However, there are many problems connected with this subject. Who should be called a sensible citizen? What are the qualifications to be a citizen of the cities? Moreover, who should be known as the citizen of a city? Citizenship is divided on three levels in our country. We elect representatives for three levels of government. First, national level, second, state level and third on city level.

We elect corporators to look after the entire development of the city - economic, social, cultural development and civic services and planning. However, this does not seem to be happening in reality.

Maybe it is because we as citizens do not think of the city as a whole? Do we elect people who are capable of thinking of the entire city or just of our group, our caste, our lane? Do the corporators we elect have knowledge of the whole city? Or are they aware merely of their ward or section? It is true that our corporators come from common people, the society, but once they are elected, they are required to think of the city as a whole. For example, how many of the representatives who promise prompt water supply are aware of the water supply of the whole city, its problems, the administrative, technical or financial sides?

Many citizens in cities today possess smart phones and tablets. Most cities have their own websites. Information regarding the Smart City is available on those sites. Several municipal corporations have tried to involve people in the project by using these websites. How many citizens had at least a cursory glance at these sites, remains a moot question. In fact, if the corporations publish details of how many people have visited the sites, it will be a mirror for citizens to assess themselves. Young people are in connection via whatsapp every minute, how many of them know about the Smart City project? Every college can also assess these facts. This will reveal how many citizens are smart in which city.

The main point is that citizens of the Smart City should possess a minimum of knowledge of their city and the corporators must possess much more information than the citizens. Citizens also should possess a minimum knowledge of the adminsitration, their civic rights and duties. If they understand how much tax is collected and how it is spent, the administration shall also be on its toes. I think ignorance of the citizens and corporators is a major block in the development of our cities. It is of great urgency to remove this block to progress towards a Smart City.

Corporators from several cities publicly complained that the administrators did not take them into confidence. But why did they expect to be invited when a smart plan was being drawn up for their own city? What prevented them from joining the effort as a corporator or even as an ordinary citizen? How many corporators obtained information of the Smart City project on their own, know all the details, think about it and discuss with people? How many of them made people aware about the proposed plans in their wards, if not their entire city? Why did they not find about other Smart Cities in the world and compare them with their city? Did they query knowledgeable people, administrators and city planners? How many citizens questioned their corporators about Smart City? The purpose behind raising these questions is that we should attempt to assess how smart we are.

We have some rights as an individual and also an opportunity to take part in governance. We are expected to create a governance system which works for the common welfare of all. No doubt, it is the municipality who should take care of the basic needs of all citizens, but citizens are also expected to contribute to the process. The basic needs of citizens can only be provided by public organizations. But when the state-owned transport system gains or loses it is every citizen who gains or loses. A bus service being run in loss cannot continue indefinitely to provide, sustainable and efficient transport.

No improvements in the service are possible. This leads to a proliferation of privately owned cars. The roads belong to everybody but are occupied by private vehicles and the sufferers are pedestrians and bus passengers.

Every citizen has the right to use public services and the responsibility to pay for it. We are highly conscious about our individual civic rights, but not equally of our common responsibilities. We are not aware of the loss to the public resources and services and that has turned us indifferent. If sustainable services is our responsibility, the publicly owned organizations must run in profit. Tolerance of the loss leads to wastage of resources, pilferage, corruption become abundant and blocks are created in qualitative improvement. Loss in public organizations is our own loot. As long as we have such shortcomings in our civic attitude, cities cannot turn smart.

It is true that smart leadership is required to create smart citizens, however, smart leadership in a democratic country can be elected only if the citizens are smart. Smart citizens first or smart leaders first remains an unanswered question!

Global Reference

In today's connected world any thought arising in one part quickly spreads all over the world. A concept like the Smart City seems fresh, appealing and easy and turns out to be the talk of common folks. However, it is not always that the majority understands all the aspects of the thought behind such ideas in depth. This is why a serious subject like Smart City is being discussed in a flippant manner. Some people are ignoring it as incomprehensible or of no consequence.

In the 1990s, much before the concept of smart city, the concept of sustainable city development never reached India. This concept of raising the living standard of not only today's citizens but also of generations to come, was taken up very seriously by a backward country like Brazil. Several cities world over have studied and attempted to bring into existence cities with emphasis on the human body, emotions and public interests of citizens. India has totally side-stepped these efforts and vaulted into the campaign of Smart City creation.

Along with the experiments for sustainable and people-oriented cities several technological experiments were conducted in developed countries.

Evolving continually they have reached an advanced stage in the smart city concept. These attempts were in the direction of making the cities more efficient, people-oriented and eco-friendly. It has been a cautious, step by step process. These experiments were conducted by mayors of cities who had been molded in the traditions of liberal, modern and worker's movements. The role played by cities' leaders in shaping the public transport system have been revolutionary. Smart city is the next step in those novel experiments.

New developing countries like Brazil have opted for strict financial planning. They had the courage to take tough decisions after consulting experts in each related field. The decisions they took were tough and unpleasant for citizens who were accustomed to private cars. These leaders took the pains of explaining such decisions to the common man to garner support. It was not easy for any of these cities to regulate private cars. Whether it was removing one channel for private cars and making it available for buses in crowded London or Curitiba or Bogota, convincing citizens was an ordeal they faced. Removing parking lots from roads was difficult in every city. Such parking lots are a hindrance to the traffic. The charges for parking are very low and it is the richer strata of the society who benefits from parking there. However, most citizens think parking on the roads is there right. To bring roads in full use it is necessary to curb the interests of some. People-oriented traffic polices are necessary to achieve this. People accustomed to use of motor cars cannot digest such a decision. These leaders had the courage to bring about a change. They had the guts to change laws to this effect and keen interest to use innovative technology. A Mumbai-based firm had helped in regulating the traffic in London. Such experiments have not been carried out in even a single city in our country. However, the economists in central ministry have first and foremost become aware of the need to improve our cities.

None of the local political leaders took any part in the Smart City Project or the previous Jawaharlal Nehru National Urban Rehabilitation project in India. The urban revival program was begun with the initiative of the prime minister and administrative officers while the political leaders were busy in power struggle. Dr. Manmohan Singh, an economist, was the prime minister then. The IIT in Mumbai had prepared an attractive vehicle for use of people in the vicinity. All that the government needed to do was to make a change in law giving importance to motor vehicles.

Local Reference

Jawaharlal Nehru National Urban Rehabilitation Project was an important program to improve our cities before the Smart City Project was mooted. The project was taken up only after the new economic policy of Liberalization, Privatization and Globalization had taken off. During this period there was growing investment at the Central level in customs, income tax and foreign investment. People has some succor as new jobs were created. Economy was growing at a higher rate for a decade and the country had benefited. Electricity and telephone services improved very quickly. However, since no solution could be found to affordable houses the issue of slums and unauthorized constructions became serious. The danger of pollution and damage to ecology reached a new high in metropolitan cities. The local administrative systems in cities became weaker. The cities went into very bad shape as they could not face the increasing problems. The local leadership was not mature enough to counter these problems. There was capable and brilliant manpower available in the cities, yet politics had managed to keep them away right since independence. Immature people living in the past glories populated the political field. Immoral persons who knew how to take disadvantage of the voting process and power had ascended in the municipalities.

Of course, there were exceptions. Chandrababu Naidu, when he was chief minister, trying to usher in many changes in Hyderabad. However, this resulted in neglect of the rural areas and he was ousted in the very next election. Citizens in Bangalore undertook studies and planning for development of Bangalore. The local information technologist and entrepreneurs took voluntary initiative. However, they were side-tracked in party politics.

The decline of Mumbai has become a worrisome subject for researchers around the world. Ample research is being conducted in universities abroad on the maladies ailing Mumbai. After much deliberation, Sarbana, a government organization from Singapore was invited by Mumbai Metropolitan Region Development Corporation to plan in a novel way for the next twenty and forty years respectively. Accordingly studies and planning was undertaken but lack of response from politicians rendered the exercise futile.

The Jawaharlal Nehru National Urban Rehabilitation Project was planned for Indian cities with a population over ten lakhs. The central government was to provide one lakh crore rupees in a time span of seven years. This aid was to be spent from improving basic services in the cities. The state government and the municipal corporation were to contribute equal amount. The total of two lakh crores were to be spent on improving water supply, sewage system, transport and affordable housing. The project was begun in 2005 and ended in 2012. The results were studied in depth and Smt. Isher Ahluwalia, an economist presented the report to the government. It is available on the Central Government's website. She also wrote a book titles *Transforming Our Cities* which is quite famous. She has recorded some novel experiments in some our cities. The subjects covered are - 1. City Planning 2. E-governance for public services 3. Water - the lifeline of cities 4. Sewage management 5. Solid Waste management 6. Urban transport system

As Isher Ahluwalia points out the tragedy is that we do not have experts to plan the cities for a vast country of one hundred and twenty five crores. The think-tank had realized this drawback as early as 2008. Experts were not available to prepare a new metropolitan plan with the Mumbai Metropolitan Corporation either considered most advanced. Smt. Ahluwalia's reported brought out the fact that this was the position with all cities in the country.

5

INDIA'S SMART CITY CAMPAIGN, 2015

The Smart City Campaign was announced in India in June 2015. This had preceded by the Loksabha elections as well as elections in some states in 2014. Mumbai, Pune and some other major cities will go to poll for municipal elections in 2017. Although the effort of JNNUR project had yielded some results in some cities, it did not help the then ruling coalition in Loksabha elections. In spite of this the new government realized that it was essential to improve our cities. This realization was very much needed. It is the primary concern of development in India where urbanization is taking place quite rapidly. The growth in urban India had accelerated the economic growth in the last two years. Cities had increased in size and population. The number of rural poor had fast decreased but there was significant rise in the number of urban poor.

A new, improved JNNUR project had been prepared by the previous central government. The new government made some changes in this and prepared the 'Smart City Project' in 2016. Such schemes cannot be launched without preparation, study and consultation.

The government had made provision of one lakh crore rupees for the JNNURP to be implemented in sixty six metropolitan cities in the country. State governments and local administrations had come up with equal funds. Basic infrastructure worth Rupees two lakh crores was expected to come up in five years. In reality the amount was not spent, the reason being the municipalities did not have the capacity to expend all the provided funds. The lacked experience to complete major projects.

Cities and Projects

The overall structure of the Smart City Project is similar to JNNURP, however, the central government is going to provide five hundred crore rupees to hundred cities to be expended over a period of five years. In addition every city and state together have to gather five hundred crore rupees in all. There is no limit of one thousand crore for projects in a city, however, the city will have to raise the extra amount needed on its own. This has led to a propaganda that the new government has provided less budget than the previous government. This is true as far as each city is concerned, however, the total number of cities has been increased. The centre is to decide how many cities in a state are to be chosen for aid under the project, but the state government has to choose the cities. The number of cities to be chosen in a state will depend on the size of the state, population and extent of urbanization. Hence, Uttar Pradesh has a maximum thirteen, Tamil Nadu twelve and Maharashtra has ten cities chosen under the Smart City Project. The chosen cities in Maharashtra are New Mumbai, Nasik, Thane, Mumbai, Amravati, Sholapur, Nagpur, Kalyan-Dombivili, Aurangabad and Pune. Those from Karnataka are Belgavi, Mangaluru, Shivamogga, Hubbali-Dharwad, Tumkuru and Davangere.

Bloomberg Philanthropy, an organization from USA is assisting the Central government in the Smart City Project. Michael Bloomberg is a multi-billionaire from the States. He had executed sustainable development plans in New York City when he was the mayor. At that time Rohit Agarwal had come up with 'Plan New York' and assisted Bloomberg to a great extent. He is a professor in the School of International and Public Affairs in Colombia University. His organization 'Side Walk' experiments in civic development. He is assisting the Smart City experiment in India. His definition of Smart City: 'improving people's lives using technology' is simple and easy to understand. His advice to the Central government is to include competitive spirit in the Smart City project. According to him, the lack of freedom to local municipalities can become a hindrance in the Smart City project. He is quite right in saying that one should not be unduly impressed by the global experiments, finding solutions for local preferences is most important in the Smart City project and city's sustainable development.

It is important to make the villages also smart in smart development. Cities are dependent for food, water and other natural products. It is necessary to see to the development of villages while developing smart cities. Smart cities cannot develop in isolation.

It is important for a city to identify which technology is affordable to its citizens and necessary for development. It is not an easy job to select from a plethora of technologies. Unfortunately, it is precisely this discretion that we lack. Couple with false pride this leads to misuse of the aid we receive. Smart City project has kindled great expectations on the local as well as global level. The danger of these expectations not getting fulfilled is even greater.

Following information about the Smart City concept is available on the central government's website. It has been presented here with the intention of making it available in a suitable form which the common citizen will find interesting and sufficient.

Restoration of problem-ridden areas:

Selecting an area of minimum five hundred square acres which is lacking in planning and basic civic services and improve it by finding smart answers to its problems.

Reconstruction of old, dangerous areas:

Reconstructing with proper planning those areas which are in a dangerous condition. Such areas should be at least fifty acres in size. It is expected that an area of slum or of old, dilapidated, thickly populated area will be selected.

Creating new colonies:

Selecting open land in growing cities and on the city's periphery to create all sorts of modern basic amenities using smart technology. The area of such a locality should be minimum two hundred fifty acres.

Cities have the option of choosing one or two or combining two of the options.

Smart Urban Services:

A project to choose any one service and making it smart for the entire city. For example water, sewage disposal, solid waste or public transport. Improving one or two of these services using smart technology. There is also a provision for a proposal to make administrative service smart. The expectation is that there should be an improvement in the entire city's service leading to an improvement in living standard of the citizens providing ring roads to the smaller cities to curb traffic from problem because of heavy vehicles.

Amrut Scheme:

Along with the Smart City Project for hundred cities, the central government declared in June 2015 a scheme to provide houses and amrut for all by the year 2022. Amrut means 'Atal Mission for Rejuvenating and Urban Transformation.' This scheme has to be implemented by the states along with 'Swacch Bharat' and other schemes. Maharashtra has selected forty two cities for the Amrut scheme, Uttar Pradesh fifty four, Tamil Nadu thirty three, Andhra Pradesh thirty one, Rajasthan thirty, West Bengal twenty eight, Bihar twenty seven, Odisha and Haryana nineteen each. Amrut Scheme aims to provide affordable housing and the supporting infrastructure in five hundred cities. Two hundred twenty five cities have already been selected out of five hundred. Central funds will be available to municipalities for this project.

Hriday Scheme:

Along with Smart City and Amrut schemes was announced yet another scheme viz. National Heritage City Development and Augmentation Yojana. Under this scheme, the central government will provided five hundred crore rupees to twelve cities. These funds are to be utilized to improve basic services in areas surrounding monuments in places of historical importance. Ajmer, Amaravati, Amritsar, Badami, Dwarika, Gaya, Kanchipuram, Mathura, Puri, Varanasi, Velankani and Warangal are the cities selected under this scheme. A city planning expert committee has been constituted to direct this scheme and its implementation overseen by a committee comprising of secretaries from various departments of the central government. In addition a committee has been constituted of administrative officers in each city. The planning and construction work will be undertaken by special experts and advisors.

Shamaprasad Mukherji Urban Mission:

This scheme was also announced along with the Smart City Project in 2015. This scheme envisaged development of cluster of villages with 25,000 to 5000 population. The state governments are expected to choose such clusters. Five thousand one hundred and forty two crore rupees have been earmarked for this project to be expended over five years. Tap water, sewerage, schools, skills development, tiny industrial complexes, agricultural processing, village roads, digital literacy, ecological protection are the various heads under which the funds are to be utilized.

Smart City Process:

The central government has provided a format for applying for the Smart City Project. Since the proposals from each city will be in a standard format, it will not be difficult to read and understand. It is mandatory for all necessary administrative bodies to be involved while preparing the proposal.

The list for providing details while submitting the Smart City proposal is very extensive. Submitting the proposal is indeed a smart task. Studying the proposals reveals considerable information about the city, its problems and the solutions suggested.

It can be seen that the officers of the city administration find it very difficult to attend to their routine duty, hence it was a great burden for them to come up with the smart city proposals in the required timeframe. Moreover, the elected representatives are totally unqualified for this work, and they are not really interested in participating in directly useful planning process. This necessitated advisory companies. These companies are Indian but some of the companies have foreign partners. They carried out the responsibility of actually preparing the application, in planning, in financial management, smart technology. Experts in engineering and social fields also contributed. These aspects are reflected in the Smart City reports, proposals and their presentation.

Every city was expected to come up with an attractive, appropriate 'logo' and a 'vision statement'. Accordingly the cities applying for the project have created their logos and vision statement. Some cities appealed to the artists and conducted a competition to suggest logos. Bhubaneshwar, Pune, Jaipur, Surat, Kochi, Ahmedabad, New Delhi, Jabalpur, Vishakhapattan, Solapur, Davangere, Indore, Coimbatore, Kakinada, Belgavi, Udaipur, Guwahati, Chennai, Ludhiana and Bhopal were the cities selected in the first list. Pune stood second and Solapur ninth in this competition. Cities have been selected from each important state and there is much difference in the population and size of these cities. However, each of these cities has a minimum population of ten to twelve lakhs.

An important condition stipulated in the project is that the Smart City should be planned through people's participation. The administrators of various cities are seen to have utilized various methods to approach the public. In Pune the daily 'Sakal' took initiative. The Pune municipal corporation involved students to feed data in computers. Mobile phone were utilized to understand public opinion. Most of the cities started their own websites for the Smart City Project. Citizens have noted air and sound pollution among one of the major concerns along with other issues.

Although many have opined that these methods are not sufficient, this was the first time people experienced such campaigns to reach them and participated enthusiastically. At least people were happy that they could participate in planning for the first time. Hitherto, people's representatives have been taking all decisions on behalf of the public. People's opinions and problems have rarely featured in the process.

This kind of people's participation is a novel experience not only for the public but for the administrators too. They will need more time to learn the art and technique of conducting such meetings with calm efficiency and put forth their points of view. Our democratic system is noisy and no one listens to another. People observe their representatives in parliament and legislatures and follow them. Everyone speaks in loud tones, they make allegations, go on in a rambling manner and the main points get lost in the process. The tradition of one person speaking and others listening uncritically is not conducive to democracy. The administrators, planners and political leaders have to make a lot of effort to understand what citizens want. Our civic and voluntary organizations are also not mature enough to participate in a responsible manner. There is no unanimity amongst them. Clever politicians can use them to their own advantage. There is much confusion about handling traffic problems. Restrictions on private cars, rates for parking, bus fares, special ways for buses and cyclists, priority to pedestrians are not understood well enough. This is natural in a way. Everyone has to learn how to abide by the opinions of the traffic expert yet take decisions in stipulated time by majority. The administration can have technical, financial and legal difficulties. They are under undue pressure from people's representatives and vested interests. Citizens have to understand this aspect. These are new facets of responsible and participatory development. Making the old village councils and municipalities pro-participatory is a great challenge. New facets of the problem are becoming visible in the Smart City project. There are bound to be differences and maturity will come out of such difference of opinion. The democratic process is long and constantly evolving one. It cannot emerge automatically but has to be inculcated in the society with some effort. Considering all the ground reality, one must say that the projects that have come up for Smart City are remarkable.

The central government has issued a logo depicting a butterfly and urban roads. The logo for Amrut scheme shows a peacock feather. Pictorial language can be used without words and meaning conveyed to the public. Preparation of logos is part of the Smart City project. The logo adopted by Pune city shows a bird in flight in many colors and with English and Marathi words. It implies manifold meanings. Several other cities have come up with multicolored, graphic symbols. Some samples of these logos can be found in this book. This pictorial language has been generated anew by cities and citizens. This was also part of the effort to involve the public.

The vision statements of several cities are also very attractive. Here are some examples:

1. Bhuwaneshwar, Odisha	Towards a smarter Bhuwaneshwar through participatory decision-making, responsible government and open access to information and technology.
2. Pune	Pune holds important place in both Maharashtra and India. It aspires to become a global urban center by offering its citizens a great quality of life.
3. Jaipur	Aspires to leverage its heritage and tourism through innovative and inclusive solutions, to enhance the quality of life.

| **4. Surat** | Providing equal access to best quality physical and social infrastructure and efficient mobility through state of the art technology. |
| **5. Kalyan-Dombivili** | To facilitate a convenient living habitat for its citizens with excellent transit facilities and enable easy access to other parts of Mumbai Metropolitan Region. |

Information about some Smart City Projects is given below. This will help to clear some doubts in the minds of readers about the Smart City Projects. If citizens understand what is going to happen in the city and what is possible, then they may feel a greater attachment to their city. People's attachment to the city must grow in order to improve the cities.

Observations:

It has been found that eleven proposals have been received for E-governance, eleven for improving traffic system, four for solid waste management, one for improving tax collections through GIS technology, one for disaster management, one for smart lights and one for basic social service. Most of the corporations has stressed on modernizing the water supply system. The funds available from Amrut Scheme will be utilized this. This means that most corporations have not succeeded in providing an efficient waster supply. There are various reasons and there are different reasons for this failure in each city. Financial investment, availability of water, transportation, distribution and waste water planning, technology, repairs and maintenance, water uses and the balancing of income and expenditure are factors responsible for this failure. One important common factor in all cities is the declining water management. The municipal administration is very backward in all these areas. Water and drainage management is one of the most crucial constitutional responsibility of municipal corporations. JNNUR project had given utmost importance to this responsibility. The central government had provided funds for this without any conditions. Most of the corporations availed the funds, but nowhere is seen its effective utilization. Water-management did improve in some cities to some extent, but the improvement was not enough. This is why most cities have once again added water management to their Smart City proposals. It is important to invest in smart meters, account of water, water supply to all parts of city and efforts to minimize leakage etc, what is of more importance is a stop to political interference. In Pune there is sufficient water and in Solapur it is insufficient, yet there is a shortfall in recovery in both places. This is a chronic ailment and it is political in nature. In Solapur the Smart City funds will be utilized to process water for use and to store rainwater and there is nothing objectionable in this proposal. Unless water supply and drainage are thought of together the management cannot be effective. However, very few corporations have combined water management with reuse. Actually concentrating only on supply of water is addressing only half the problem. Such planning is useless from the point of view of sustainable development. There is a dire need for public toilets and it has been almost universally neglected. Unless the organizational and administrative structure is fundamentally changed the water supply cannot become smart in any of the municipal corporations.

Traffic is another important subject which is troubling all cities. The exponential growth of privately owned vehicles, roads broadened by sacrificing footpaths and vehicles parked on roads are common experiences yet not even one city has demonstrated readiness to take up a unified traffic policy. The reason being traffic is not a technical but political problem. Unless political influence is removed there can be smartness in traffic. Smart traffic can come about only by a combination of technology, planning and management.

The real culprits for the deterioration of cities are the state governments. The piled up mistake after mistake instead of correcting the faulty policies of the 1960s. The central government had advised all state governments to draw up traffic policies. Prototype of a model system had also been provided.

The most important aspect of Smart City project from a political point of view is that of forming a special company. All projects in this scheme are going to be conducted under a special company. The company will be responsible for all matters from planning to execution. Once the project is completed all the smart mechanisms will be under the possession of the municipal corporation.

Information system has to be always active and continually updated in case of modern, smart traffic and other services. This will not be an easy task for the existing mechanism of the corporations. No scheme can be successful in the long term, unless co-operation is extended by the staff. Several cities purchased excellent buses from the JNURP funds, but they lack funds to carry out repairs, maintenance and spare parts. One might afford to purchase the latest computer-system and information technology but it is quite expensive to keep them operative. It is a common experience that medical equipment in government hospitals costing crores of Rupees are inoperative more time than not. Moreover, trained and skilled manpower to operate systems is expensive. Appointments are not timely. By the time staff is appointed, machines lie idle and go out of order. Smart machines are sensitive and have to be used with much care. The problem with smart technology is not only financial it is more about intelligent, responsible and efficient manpower.

Improving the traffic in selected areas will be one of the most important task under the Smart City project. All the other services are located underneath the roads, they have to be arranged for before the roads are built. Footpaths and bicycle paths come up last. Citizens need to understand all these matters from experts. The construction should be carefully watched. Organizations like BRT should be supported with proper understanding. This necessitates that the politicians craze for flyovers needs to be curbed. Among the twenty cities chosen for Smart City project, fifteen have chosen to reconstruct old areas. Two cities have chosen tourism and one has chosen natural resources.

A number of technologies of varying size and costs are available for converting waste/garbage to fertilizer or energy. However, these smart technologies need smart citizens to adopt them. Not a single city has thought of educating citizens to bifurcate organic and non-organic waste or to educate them to keep roads free of garbage. If the citizens and their representative corporators are opposed to such a scheme the administrators will prove ineffective. Some proposals include a combination of Swacch Bharat and other schemes with the Smart City project, however, not a single corporation has come up with a campaign for public toilets. They have given no thought to it at all. In reality, this is a very serious problem and it can be solved through the co-operation of voluntary organizations and citizens.

The other most important and difficult problem is that of slum areas, but not one city corporation has proposed a scheme to tackle it. Probably the administrative officers and those living in proper houses do not consider it as a problem at all. The viewpoint of citizens living in most cities is faulty. Most think that the people living in slum areas are responsible for problems of water supply or the squalor in the city. The urban middle class is lacking in humanism and tolerance. They would prefer to chase them away than improve the slum localities of the underprivileged. It is also a fact that slums come up because of political gains. Since there is no thought of providing a small house with smart services to everyone the subject has simply not appeared in the Smart City program. Affordable housing is a local issue and city corporations are not shouldering any responsibility in that respect. Unless the state governments change their policies no solution for this predicament can be found.

Smart electricity is relatively simple issue and is beneficial from the point of environment, energy and financial savings. We will see solar energy used more and more in the coming decades as the production costs are going down. Just as smart phones became cheaper it will be possible to produce solar energy in homes and make them self-sufficient. Any surplus energy generated can be distributed to needy sectors of the city through power supply grids. These days electricity is generated in households in a states like California which have abundant sunshine. Larger companies and factories are installing solar panels atop their plants, yards, parking lots etc. Cities can take up several novel projects taking advantage of solar or non-traditional energy sources. However, none of the city corporations have shown the far-sightedness and innovativeness. In fact, there are very few experiments to embrace modern technology which will become foundations for the sustainable city concept. There will be the odd successful experiment. It will be useful to an extent, however, nothing glorious, magnificent or noble is perceived in the Smart City proposals.

There are two factors necessary for the success of the Smart City, about which there is much apprehension. Smart administration and smart citizens are the two factors. The paths to make them smart are quite different. There are many facets of smart administration and unless each of these created consciously the administration will not become smart. There are at least three factors necessary for smart administration – first is having a clear goal, second is the means needed to attain the objective and third is the motivation and dedication of the managers to achieve the goals. We rarely come across such inspiration in today's administrative system. And where it exists, there are attempts to destroy it. The same kind of indifference is seen among citizens. Citizens are ready to spend any amounts for buying gadgets for personal pleasure, but there is not tendency on the part of citizens to spend for the common interest.

Evaluation:

Some years back the Gujarat government started a grand scheme known as 'GIFT city' (Gujarat International Finance Tee-City). It is now called as 'Gift Smart City'. This dreamland is coming up on seven hundred acre land on the banks of the river in Ahmedabad and Gandhi Nagar. One can see the information, advertisement and attractive pictures of this scheme on the internet. Bullet train has recently been announced between Ahmadabad and Mumbai. This could be an attempt to connect the Gift Smart City to Mumbai's financial centers to generate competition. Many a time schemes are conceived bypassing the public and without a dialogue with them. The media is roped in or their independence encroached upon. People have to be alert to this danger. Although the Smart City campaign has evolved through the combination of JNNURP and Smart City, it seems to be under the shadow of Gift City concept. I remembered Jane Jacob's words while browsing through the Gift City mission pictures. She says, "It is easy to draw pictures of a dream city, however, to rejuvenate a living, vibrant city needs resolution."

Advertisements can mislead people and a political race on mega projects is begun. The desire to bring about change with small changes is affected and the ultimate loser is the common man. People are bombarded with gleaming advertisements out of nowhere. This happens through the undue ambitions, impractical political daredevilry and grandiose daydreaming.

The Smart City experiment in India has begun without proper cultivation of the society, the ground and people's mindset. Although mentioned in the JNNURP review no efforts have been made to end the dearth of trained human resources for this purpose. On top of it the city administrators are burdened with the responsibility of the Smart City project.

Chances of Success:

From the above discussion readers will gather how difficult is the path of Smart City Projects. If chances are to be estimated, a twenty to forty percent success may be expected in some cities similar to the JNNURP scheme. Those cities which have capable administrators, politicians support to a special company and participation of local people will be able to utilize the opportunity. If this happens, it can be treated as a limited success of the

Smart City Project. It remains to be seen where and how the handling of the project by a special private company succeeds or is allowed to succeed. My guess is that the new company may succeed, at least for some time, better than the existing local administration in most cities. The chances of the company succeeding will be more if the local citizens help and co-operate with the company and supervise its work. Whether the persons heading those companies are effective will depend on their skills.

There is one more scale to measure the success of the Smart City project. It needs to be measured how the local municipal workers utilize the opportunity and get trained. The private advisory companies will learn a lot from this experience and gain financially too. The city corporations can learn to be self-sufficient. Some companies may create new technologies and make it part of their operations. They can adopt foreign technology and methods to suit the local conditions. This experience will help them to create new concepts and techniques. It will be an achievement of the Smart City project if the participating citizens, administrators and officers of the private company become more thoughtful, wise and innovative. Some local organizations, professional city planners and social workers can participate and give a new direction to small towns.

There is yet another hurdle in the path of this grand scheme – that of the citizens not being smart. An even more hurdle is that of the corporators not being smart. The people's representatives in the municipalities are only worried about their vote bank. All they know of public service is planting a few trees here and there in their wards, erecting a few benches, or constructing a public toilet or fountain or ugly sculptures. They achieve this within the limit of a few lakh rupees and feel proud. They are not even aware of the problems of their entire ward and the problems of the city as a whole are beyond their comprehension. An exception to this only goes on to prove the rule. The Smart City Project has not even touched the surface of this problem. That is why probably the corporators have been kept away from the Smart City show. After the corporators have expressed dissatisfaction over this, may be the mayor and a couple of members will be added to the team in the Special Company, however, their role will be a minor one. In contrast the role of the commissioner and the newly appointed special executive officer will have the control of the Smart City project in the city. The commissioners of most municipal corporations are selected intelligent cadre from the Indian

Administrative Service. They are graduates from medicine, engineering, art or science. Whatever educational background they may have come from they are well trained in managing the various departments of government. They are young, experienced, keen and ambitious. They are duty-bound to complete the task assigned to them. However, they may not be creative enough to come up with innovative ideas for city planning. Not all commissioners are capable of grasping new technology and systems and accepting them.

Since cities under the Smart City program have been selected competitively, in a sense it is a competition among the commissioners. Most of the commissioners have exerted and done much work in a short time. In this short period they have not only studied the problems of their city but also thought about solutions. They have worked with advisors who are experts in city planning, layout, basic services, traffic and financial management. It is the commissioners who have presented the proposal to local citizens as well as the committee in Delhi. One can view the presentation made to citizens on you tube. These presentations reveal the skills of the commissioner. The presence of the mayor and corporators at such presentations seems cursory.

Elected mayors of various cities participate in the global discussion on Smart City. They speak authoritatively on the problems facing their city. Their emotional commitment to and responsibility towards the city is palpable in their voice, in their presentation.

Many citizens of our cities are not even aware as to who is the mayor of their city and most of the mayors are not aware of the problems faced by their citizens. The reason for this is hidden in the political race and mentality behind capturing the mayor's seat. The mentality, thinking and crass behavior of people's representatives is feudal in essence. Even where the power is with communists they too are taken by the helicopter culture. Moreover, the socialist and communists do not appear to be caring for the global view while thinking of cities and urbanization. Today there is a dearth of leaders who are genuinely aware of the local city's problems, and capable of independently thinking about the complicated issues. We do not come across such leaders in Maharashtra or anywhere in India. The letter 'S' in Smart denotes Specific. Every city is specific hence the policy cannot be understood by parties and people thinking in a wholesale or bookish manner. Cities are liberating and generous.

The Smart City Project has revealed the gap between the administration and elected representatives in terms of authority and responsibility.

The colonial rulers used to say, "Indians are not capable of modern administration." Although the administration at the centre and state levels is not ideal, it is independent and self-sufficient that is why the country is undivided.

Luckily, there is not much opposition as yet to the Smart City project from social and voluntary organizations. There are two possible reasons for this. First is that the workers' and citizens' movements which were always taking opposing postures have been weakened. And the few organizations that are still functional do not appear to care much about the intentions, complications and technology behind the Smart City project. A minor opposing voice is that of the handful of leaders from established political parties, however, that does not seem to be strong enough. None of the leadership in established political parties have taken a stance opposite the Smart City project. The Smart City project in Mumbai seems to have fizzled out without much ado. The Marathi corporators are opposed to making Mumbai a Smart city and the New Mumbai municipality has openly opposed the Smart city project. The leaders of New Mumbai think that theirs is a well-planned city and they are capable and smart enough to sort out their own problems. Their contention is true to an extent. That is why the local representatives are averse to the interference from state and central government under the pretext of Smart city project.

The corporate sector companies involved in advisory role in Smart City project are its staunch supporters. They are its beneficiaries too. They had played a major role in the previous JNURP. Each selected city has received two crore rupees for studying and planning under the Smart City project. The advisory companies have been active in this. Young generation trained in civic planning and management field are participating in this activity. They are being guided by some experienced experts from abroad. There is much competition in the field. City planning was a highly neglected field until now. Planners used to be employed only in government sector. For the first time they are being offered important jobs in private sector under the Smart City project. Renowned Indian and global companies in information field are also supporting the project. These companies are eager for financial and executive participation. Multinationals like IBM, Cisco, Siemens from the IT sector do not aim merely to sell smart city technology, their real profit will come in from maintaining the advanced systems in smart cities. The initial investment in hardware is important, but even more important for these companies is the repairs and maintenance and intellectual skill involved in continual growth. Their real investment is their long-sightedness and smart marketing skills. No doubt, local, trained personnel will gain employment in future and new local capabilities will arise. Local entrepreneurs will be created in future to provide smart services to other cities. That is why many national and international companies are viewing the central government's Smart City project with great hopes.

As of today one cannot presume whether the Smart City campaign will succeed or fail entirely. However, it does not seem likely that it will garner many points and succeed in several cities. The objective of this book is not to predict the future of the Smart City project. There is much curiosity about the project among all strata of people. Even citizens from poor localities are welcoming the scheme and their main question is, 'what will be our place in the project?' 'Will we be considered in the project or not?' It is more important to respond to the curiosity of the citizens, provide information and demonstrate the opportunities and risks. It is necessary to keep alive this interest. I hope this book will assist in keep the interest alive and make the citizens aware of not only their rights but responsibilities too.

Will cities in India become smart?

No one will disagree on the need for improvement in our cities. However, it is better not to harbor illusions about the Smart City Project that it will overnight turn our cities as smart as cities in the West. Several cities have used pictures of tall rise buildings with glass fronts, flyovers and metros in their visions. Citizens should not let themselves be lured by such visuals. If we can make our cities a little better instead of totally smart, that will be an achievement in itself. At the same time one should avoid ridiculing the Smart City project. Just it is wrong to harbor unrealistic expectations it is also wrong to despise or counter any attempt at improvement. A realistic answer to the question, 'whether Indian cities will become smart?', can be, 'some cities might improve to some extent.' If citizens become smart along with cities, it might be a more sustainable benefit.

BELGAVI: THE SMART CITY

Vision

Belagavi, a thousand year old city with a rich heritage and a mosaic of different communities has a vision of an "inclusive, livable, culturally vibrant city emerging as an eminent destination for health, education, ancillary industry and logistics sectors". (HEAL City).

We envisage optimum livable atmosphere to our citizens. Developing on pulsating hubs of health, education and also leveraging the potential human resource with skill development, planned industrial area development, attracting investment towards ancillary and logistics sectors growth.

We also envisage a city where an efficient transportation system allows us to access our places of work, recreation or entertainment speedily, a city that is relatively safe, a city which protects its heritage sites and parks, a city which constantly strives to lower its carbon footprint by harnessing renewable and which cares for, and lives in harmony with its environment.

We envisage inclusive livability by comprehensive infrastructure development through convergence also provisioning adequate revenue generation leveraging on innovative use of potential and viable space with ULB.

We also envisages that cultural vibrancy will be kept intact through model preservation activities of Fort heritage structure, heritage park, lakes and also citizens engagement with his city through walkability.

From city profile it is derived that the level of basic infrastructure is uneven with spatial variations across the city and there is need for providing the same evenly to entire population Hence providing quality infrastructure and universal coverage is envisaged.

Overall aspirations and goals for city are derived from feedback obtained from extensive and credible citizen engagement across all sectors of the society.

GOALS

Belagavi has set out for itself a calibrated path that will make it a highly livable city with time bound comprehensive infrastructure development.

Quantifiable Goals:

- 24x7 Potable water for all assuring quality, quantity and service by 2019 with smart metering and e-billing.

- Full coverage of UGD network with sewage treatment plant, recycling and reuse of treated water by 2019 also ensuring 100 % coverage of individual and 150 public toilets.

- Assured continuous electricity supply by augmenting 12% through renewable energy also aiming at reduction of T&D losses by under ground HT&LT lines by 2019, retrofitting of existing street lights with LED to minimize energy consumption by 2017.- Achieve 100% door to door collection, segregation, scientific treatment and disposal ensuring waste to energy by 2017.

- Ensuring Intelligent Transport System assured last mile connectivity. Also ensuring of a city and 8 satellite bus terminii by 2019.

- Assured hassle free urban mobility, by completing 4 ROBs, 3 flyovers, under passes, junction improvement, pathway improvement, multi-level parking, dedicated parking zones and also ensuring safety and security through E-surveillance and police by 2018.

- Development of cycle tracks, improvement of footpath for walkability by completing 407 and 702 km by 2017 respectively.

- Ensuring the CDP of 2014 implemented with issue of building permissions mandating solar rooftop panels aiming towards provisioning for green building by 2018 along with already mandated rain water harvesting and solar water heaters.

- Achieve 80% coverage of flat roofed government buildings with Solar PV Panels by 2018.

- Ensuring air quality, maintaining desired green cover, developing parks and open spaces, water bodies by 2018.

- Provisioning adequate housing stock to EWS and slum dwellers through integrated vertical development by unlocking the reserved land of 30 acres by 2018.

- CNG and PNG Gas access to domestic, commercial and industrial use of the city by year 2018.

- ICT enablement by creating centralized command center and E-Governance to be fully accomplished through "Belagavi One Center" across the city. Providing 28 services of the ULB by 2017 and 72 services, including processing, to be online by 2018, with all 144 services by 2020.

- Preserving rich heritage Fort structure, developing heritage park with available 160 acres there by promoting cultural history to enable value based growth by 2018.

- New 18 km commercial corridor and Construction of Multi Utility Centers to augment decentralized growth, revenue recovery and promoting mixed land use at Five locations by year 2018.

- Attaining desired infrastructure levels in recreational and sports activities by constructing Art Gallery, Museum, Exhibition center, Yoga and meditation centers.

- Making available non motorized streets, walkability, network connectivity and paratransit transport by year 2017.

- Ensuring imparting desired skill sets to potential human resource viz. professionals, organized, an unorganized sectors through various skill development cecenters proposed at Five Multi-Utility Facilitation centers there by ensuring employment and sectoral growth.

Development Strategy:

Over the past five years our strategy for development of Belagavi is based on the Robust citizen engagement programme which took place over the years, by which it was mandated that we converge various development schemes for infrastructure development in the city and also leveraging on potential sectors to ensure economic growth, viability and employment.

24 x 7 water supply scheme, implementation of the master plan, Under Ground Cabling works, planning and clearance for UGD system and development of ten water bodies, rejuvenation of open wells, construction of RoB, pedestrian underpass was the result of the citizen engagement and were implemented on the basis of aspirations of the citizens.

Now it is our strategy to extend our approach further on the basis of recent reengagement of the citizens to cover the comprehensive and integrated infrastructure dvelopment in following areas;

Drawing upon our experience over past 5 years in the two demo zones, where the per capita consumption of water has dropped from 105 lpcd to 85 lpcd., we are upscaling the 24x7 metered water supply to the whole city with upgradation with smart meters and e-billing.

We are planning for Sewerage network for uncovered Areas and a Sewage Treatment Plant for the entire city with reusage of treated sewage water for industries.

We are planning for Multi Utility Centers with Green building concepts for innovative use of open spaces available. These MUCs will act as new public services centers under one umbrella, impetus to the economic development of surrounding areas and also acts as a revenue generating model for ULB.

As part of our strategy we are having plans for protection of water bodies in the city and also beautifications of their surroundings and develop tourism and recreational areas. For rejuvenation of water bodies all primary and secondary storm water drains are planned.

Hence it is proposed to develop the water body or the moat around the fort and the pertinent area as heritage park. Within the fort a district museum is proposed. The ancient temples and mosques inside the fort are to be properly showcased.

The strategy is to develop 18 Km stretch of potential commercial corridor generating 7% of total ABD area for the commercial activity.

153 acres of wooded land was preserved by a govt order of 2001 as heritage park and botanical garden. Plan has been developed in consultation with SPA, Delhi in 2013 for conservation of this area. To showcase the rich culture of belagavi area new art, drama.

STRATEGIC FOCUS AND CONCEPT.

Belagavi is already having a landfill site with compost plant facility. The strategy is to develop 100% segregation at source, upgrade the compost plant facility and develop a waste to energy plant for reduction of solid waste.

Emphasis is on renewable energy both solar and wind power, we are planning for solar roof top power generation of 30 MW and wind power plant of 30 MW augmenting the power requirement upto 20% by renewable energy by year 2020.

Belagavi is also getting the CNG and PNG sources for commercial and domestic distribution from year 2016 which enables using the cleaner fuel for environmental protection.

We are planning for UG cabling of HT and LT for energy efficiency. We are conserving the energy by providing LED automatic streetlights.

Our focus is on ICT enablement to bring in maximum utilization of infrastructure. Our focus is on e-governance which will have websites for public access on government services. This enables the processes on web and through smart phone applications for municipality services, property registration, tax payment and department request and information. Initially 28 services will be covered.

Using of ICT for intelligent transport system and improvement of mobility for entire city and monitoring of Air Quality is another thrust area.

The strategy is to develop a revenue generating model for recovering the O&M cost of all the proposals in Smart City.

Outer ring road is also planned around Belagavi city to decongest the city and with a view of compact development and densification in the city with beltway development within ring road.

Our other strategic focus for transforming Belagavi is to harness traditional model of development of farm to fork economy model with cold storage and processing facilities, developing seri culture, development of mechanized dairy units by encouraging entrepreneurs.

BELGAVI - MY CITY SMART CITY

SMART CITY: BELGAVI 2016-2017
SMART CITIES WITH FOCUS ON INCLUSIVE GENDER
EMPOWERMENT:

The critical analysis suggests that focus for smart city should be initially for the following four points before any large scale investments be made

1. **Smart City needs Smart People: -** A smart city needs to be made smarter or at least maintained smart. The first basic necessity is to train our citizens to be smart viz, their responsibility towards handling of garbage, traffic sense, and the entire civic sense as a whole to protect the costly infrastructure built up during the process of making the city into a smart city. This can be achieved by the following modes:

    a. **Smart Cities Readiness Workshops**: These workshops should be part of every corporator's work profile. School students, youth, professionals, women must attend these workshops at ward level.
    b. **Smart city social media:** Citizens must take initiative to upload pictures/ inform authorities through the social media about any deviations or destruction caused to facilities.
    c. **Citizens' initiative to play vigilante:** empowered citizen groups can be created to keep vigil on the maintainance of the infrastructure with help from the government

2. **Need for Periodic Maintenance: -** A Smart City involves a huge investment of over Rs 1000 Crores and it is a common knowledge that the periodic maintenance of the infrastructure created is non existing E.g.

The RPD college road was widened with Footpath and Street Lights, Road Dividers, Plantation of Trees, but the agony is that the footpaths are not fit for the pedestrians since it is uneven and shrunk in many places, the street lamps are not functioning, cables are exposed in many places and the road condition is very bad. Huge amount has been spent on this infrastructure but the periodic maintenance is non -existing. If the same continues, the entire hard earned tax payer's money in the smart city will go down the drains.

So special provisions to be made for regular annual maintenance so that the smart city could be maintained for at least 30 years hence. A good example for the above point could be the maintenance of the NH-4 Stretch from Belagavi to Kagal which is built by Punj Lloyd and maintained by Asoka Infra Projects Ltd.

Pruning trees, watering plants, repairing loose pavement tiles, covering potholes and damaged roads, etc. must be immediately done. The Corporator plays a major role in this and must be monitored by citizens groups.

No pitholes, digging of roads and damaging of property must be allowed at any cost. Any private company desirous to do must be allowed at a single point in time and any further work needs to be repaired to the original with heavy levy of penalty.

3. **Toilets for Men and Women:** - The focus area is to have smart toilets in smart city. The city corporation had built many pay-and-use toilets at important locations but unfortunately due to bad maintenance as mentioned in point no 2. all the toilets are not usable. And more importantly, there are no toilets for ladies who have to resort to seeking help at private hospitals, complexes and other places unsafe and unhygienic for them. Hence to call our city smart, we need smart toilets. Charging a minimal amount can be the best option. These toilets must be cleaned regularly and refilled with water several times a day.

   Citizens must be trained that toilets are to be kept clean by the users and it is not the responsibility of the cleaning staff.

   These toilet blocks must be provided at key places, including vegetable markets, cizty centers, near educational institutions, bus stands, railway stations, etc.

4. **Scientific Disposal of Garbage**: - Several tonnes of wet and dry garbage is generated in Belgaum city every day. This garbage is currently together dumped at Turmuri depot which is creating health hazard for the people of that area. Daily collection of garbage from homes, depositing at nodal centers and then plying trucks to this depot is a costly affair. Also, the staff on these vehicles have to work in inhuman conditions, many times smearing themselves in hazardous chemicals and fumes.

The garbage generated in the city can be processed or recycled within the city limits at very nominal prices compared with the money spent for transporting the same for long distances. To convert the bio degradable waste, use of latest technology and machines. Details as per annexure Citizens must be thoroughly trained in garbage segregation. Posters, awareness drives, animation films, prizes for cleanest wards, etc. can be constituted.

School kids must be encouraged to use these methods at home
Neighborhood citizen vigils can also be encouraged.

5. **Managing the Commercial Hub**: - Belgaum's Commercial Hub comprising of Kirloskar Road, RamdevGalli, MarutiGalli, Khade Bazaar, BasavanGalli, SamadeviGalli, GanapatGalli, and all the Bye-Lanes connecting these are the main commercial areas. Designating this area into a no- vehicle zone will encourage pedestrians to keep their vehicles at home and come for purchasing by city transport. Providing three multi layers parking at three places namely 1. Bogarves, 2. Channamma Circle & near CBT will enable the shop owners to park their vehicle near their workplace. Plan for tram lines/battery operated busses and cycle pools.

Placing dustbins, color coded garbage bins, covered rain water drains, etc. can make this quadrangle a dream to move about. Shop owners must be made to dispose their papers, cardboards, wrapping papers, etc. in designated areas only or a separate truck can collect the same every day.

A dedicated Tram line on the roadside will enable shoppers as well as owners to hop-on-hopp-off from their homes to this commercial hub without using private vehicles.

Penalizing citizens for bringing private cars to the commercial hub by levying heavy parking fee and /or entry fee at the entrance can prove a deterrent.

6. **Constructing the Ring Road**: - Connecting NH-4 Pune – Bengaluru to NH-4A Belagavi-Panaji. Connecting NH-4A to Vengurla Road and NH-4 (via Peranwadi, Vijay Nagar to Kangrali). This will encourage unconnected vehicles with Belagavi city to pass by without traffic hassles.

    Currently, all vehicles from the PB road who have to go to Goa/Sawantwadi enter the city even though they have no reason for the same.

    A ring road shall save time, effort and fuel on a large scale.

7. **Fly-Overs**: - Minimum 4 fly overs to be planned in the city on old P.B Road, Kapileshwar Road (in progress), Existing Railway overbridge to be made four lane, and between 2nd and 3rd Railway Gate. Fly overs allow seamless traffic flow to various points without vehicles having to accumulate at traffic signals. Also, they are less accident prone due to lesser traffic burden, save time, fuel and money for the nation.

    The area below the fly overs can be used, as is done at other places, for parking or for smaller commercial establishments.

8. **Maintenance of lung spaces**: - Belagavi city is fortunately blessed with a few lung spaces in the form of Vaccine Institute in Tilakwadi, Fort Defense Land and Cantonment Area. Similar large lung Spaces be provided in all new extension areas where 10 -15 acres of Forest areas be planned.

    Belgaum has some really large parks which are currently not being developed for the flora. Planting new trees with deep foliage, keeping a variety in the species, watering the trees daily, encouraging students to plant trees on birthdays, preparing seed balls and distributing as gifts, etc. can be done to involve citizens in the green drive.

    Homes with trees can be encouraged to plant more and to maintain existing ones.

    Reduction in taxes can be thought about for industries who plant and maintain trees.

    Felling of any tree must be a punishable offence unless it causes danger to human life.

9. **Sewage Water Treatment**: - 100% of sewage water be processed on lines with the technologies being adopted in Singapore and other world class cities. This water can be reused for watering the plants on public spaces,

refilling public toilets and other cleaning purposes. Industries can also avail of this water at a discounted cost for industrial purposes.

Industries treating their own water can be incentivized.

10. **Underground Cabling**: - Citizens are happy with the initiations taken by the HESCOM for laying underground cables for HT lines. The same may be adopted for LT lines.

    Citizens and Industries keep digging the road for every purpose, big and small. Hence, not only does the public infrastructure get spoilt, but a lot of agony is caused to common public and especially small children and the elderly.

    Roads get 80% of a city's budget. That's because in addition to ferrying us, they are the conduits for most utilities such as water, sewage, power, gas and phone lines. The BharatiyaJanata Party (BJP) government cleared TenderSURE (Specifications for Urban Roads Execution), or what will likely be the template for future Indian road design, in 2012, and the present Congress state government is seeing the idea through. This Rs.110-crore project (or Rs.2 crore a travel lane where 60% of the cost is for the underground utilities) covers seven busy roads in Bengaluru's central business district. The same plan can be adopted for Belgaum.

    These are roads that will require NO DIGGING once they have been laid. These companies don't need to dig—they can just slide their cables through ducts provided especially for them under these beautifully re-engineered roads.

11. **Shifting of Wholesale Vegetable Market** – The long pending issue of shifting of wholesale vegetable market may be taken up on top priority by overcoming the legal aspects in the project.

    Currently, the market clogs the city's main area that connects the bus stand to the southern and western part of the city. With trucks, pick-up vans, carts and rickshaws cramming into that area to load and offload the gunny bags, added to it the road divider which has been erected without the road being widened, causes heavy traffic jams as the vehicles pile up.

    The trash from this market is dumped on the road side or into the moats of the Belgaum fort which is declared a Heritage site. All this can be avoided if the market is shifted elsewhere, on the lines of the fruit market.

12. **Solar Roof Tops:** - Elon Musk in the US through his company Solarcity, and several other people have made use of Solar Panels set up on private and public buildings. The electricity generated therein can be shared by the owner of the building and the remaining can be pushed into the state's grid.

13. **Creating an Empowered Women's Group (EWG):** - Local areas can have EWGs of selected/chosen women of that area who can monitor the safety of the girls and women in their area. In case of some untoward incident coming to their notice, these members of the EWG can alert the police immediately.

    At a primary level, they can reprimand or tackle situations on their own. This shall be possible only with training and reinforcement among citizens.

14. **Creation of Healthcare and Wellness centers for women:** - These can beat Ward levels and accessible only by women of that area. A small subscription can be charged for the same to use the facilities which can be built on B-O-T basis with PPP model. Many women fail to exercise merely due to non-availability of time/resources/ functional areas where she finds herself comfortable. With women's diseases on the rise, these facilities are a must for any smart city to claim the tag.

What does a Smart City do?

It:

- ✓ Builds
- ✓ Operates
- ✓ Moves
- ✓ Saves
- ✓ Uses Energy
- ✓ Communicates
- ✓ Cures
- ✓ Cares
- ✓ Eats
- ✓ Exercises
- ✓ Cleans and..............LIVES SMARTLY.
- ✓ Rests

APPENDIX

1. List of 20 Smart Cities in 1st phase

1. Bhubaneswar,
2. Pune,
3. Jaipur,
4. Surat,
5. Kochi,
6. Ahmedabad,
7. Jabalpur,
8. Visakhapatnam,
9. Solapur,
10. Davangere,
11. Indore,
12. New Delhi (NDMC),
13. Coimbatore,
14. Kakinada,
15. Belgaum,
16. Udaipur,
17. Guwahati,
18. Chennai,
19. Ludhiana,
20. Bhopal

2. Total list of cities choosen for smart cities.

1. Agra
2. Ahmedabad
3. Aizawl

4. Ajmer
5. Aligarh
6. Allahabad
7. Amravati
8. Amritsar
9. Aurangabad
10. Bareilly
11. Bhagalpur
12. Bhopal
13. Bhubaneshwar
14. Biharsharif
15. Chandigarh
16. Chennai
17. Coimbatore
18. Dahod
19. Delhi
20. Dharamshala
21. Dindigul
22. Diu
23. Erode
24. Faridabad
25. Ghaziabad
26. Greater Hyderabad
27. Greater Mumbai
28. Guwahati
29. Gwalior
30. Haldia
31. Hubballi-Dharwad
32. Indore
33. Jabalpur
34. Jaipur
35. Jhansi
36. Kalyan Dombivali
37. Kanpur
38. Karnal
39. Kochi

40. Kohima
41. Kota
42. Lucknow
43. Madurai
44. Mangaluru
45. Moradabad
46. Muzaffarpur
47. Nagpur
48. Namchi
49. Nashik
50. Panaji
51. Pasighat
52. Port Blair
53. Pune
54. Raipur
55. Rampur
56. Raurkela
57. Sagar
58. Saharanpur
59. Salem
60. Satna
61. Shivamogga
62. Silvassa
63. Solapur
64. Surat
65. Thane
66. Thanjavur
67. Thoothukudi
68. Tiruchirapalli
69. Tirunelveli
70. Tiruppur
71. Tumakuru
72. Udaipur
73. Ujjain
74. Vadodara
75. Varanasi
76. Vellore